RESCUE THE DOCTOR

*What Doctors Urgently Need to Know
About the New World of Health Care*

By

DR. PETER P. PRAMSTALLER, M.D.

and

MATT SMITH

with

JEREMY BLACHMAN

Copyright © 2014 by Dr. Peter Pramstaller, Matt Smith, and Jeremy Blachman

ISBN Reserved

Layout and Design: Cheryl Perez, www.yourepublished.com

All rights reserved under International and Pan-American Copyright Conventions. No part of this book may be reproduced or transmitted in any form or by any means, electronic or mechanical, including but not limited to photocopying, electronic mail, recording or by any information storage or retrieval system—except in the case of brief quotations embodied in critical articles or reviews—without permission in writing from the copyright holder.

TABLE OF CONTENTS

Reframe *1*

Translate *61*

Deliver *103*

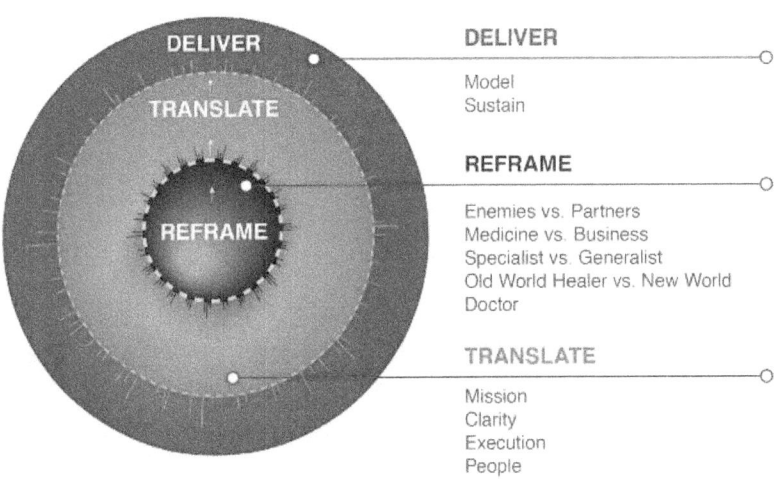

RESCUE THE DOCTOR

DELIVER

Model
Sustain

REFRAME

Enemies vs. Partners
Medicine vs. Business
Specialist vs. Generalist
Old World Healer vs. New World Doctor

TRANSLATE

Mission
Clarity
Execution
People

PREFACE

"Could [doctors] come together to overthrow the current order — to start a movement to, say, Occupy Medicine? If they did, what would be the unifying cry? Down with health insurers? Tort reform or bust? Or would it begin by expressing the thing that is most precious to them that has been lost: the opportunity to practice medicine in a way that is worthy of their dedication and love. Reclaiming a sense of meaning in medicine could be the first step to rescuing the profession."[1]

— The New York Times, "Who Will Heal The Doctors?"

---

[1] http://opinionator.blogs.nytimes.com/2013/10/02/who-will-heal-the-doctors/

This is not another book about the health care system.

This is not another book filled with buzzwords, talking about reform and reinvention, about delivering care more efficiently and more effectively, about cost control, or about checklists, filled with tools no one needs and exercises no one would ever do, the kind of book that a doctor might pick up but quickly realize isn't truly aimed at him, the individual. Sure, those kind of books might be useful, in a theoretical sense, and they certainly might make for an interesting read — we've certainly read our share of them — but they're not truly changing a doctor's day-to-day life.

This isn't a book about health care policy, or for a doctor to see what might happen, what could happen, or what should happen. This is a book to help every doctor understand what *is* happening — to him and to his colleagues — and to help everyone who works with doctors understand why doctors behave the way they do. This is a book that finally explains what is causing the uneasiness that too many doctors are feeling these days, the stress, the uncertainty, the loss of control. And then this is a book that shows you, the doctor, what you can do to empower yourself, expand the influence you have, make a real difference in your professional life, every day, and rescue yourself — and ultimately, rescue the entire profession — from the forces that are working against you.

This is a book that exists because one doctor started to realize that the professional life he thought he had signed up for didn't match the reality.

Like all doctors, Peter was trained to be a clinician — but in today's world, where doctors aren't the *lone healers* of the past but part of a much larger, much more complicated system, clinical skills aren't enough.

Peter saw his colleagues grow frustrated and start to disengage.

He saw health care slipping away from the most critical people in the system: the doctors.

He saw that the human aspect of medicine — the people — was in many ways just as important as the medicine itself.

And so Peter went on a decade-long journey to find the wisdom he needed to thrive. This book is a result of that journey, an explanation of the world doctors are living in and a set of skills to enable every doctor to cope.

If you're a doctor, you're likely starting from a place of uncertainty. You're feeling disconnected from what brought you to medicine, but you're not quite sure why. This book is designed to better help you see the current health care landscape, give you the skills to move from the Old World mindset to the New World that the profession has become, and then enable you to achieve real change — for you and for your organization.

It's a three-step plan —

Reframe the way you see the current state of health care and the huge changes affecting doctors worldwide,

Translate these industry shifts into the skills that you as doctors need in order to succeed and thrive, and then

Deliver real results.

All together, helping you become a more fulfilled, more satisfied, more successful doctor — a *rescued* one.

If you're not a doctor, but you rely on doctors to help you effectively do your job, as an administrator or other professional, we want to rescue you, too, and help you work with doctors as productively as possible. We want to explain to you why doctors are struggling, and how you can all move ahead as partners instead of enemies.

If you're a medical student, or a resident or fellow, not yet in practice, you're ahead of the game. You'll want to read this book to better understand the world you're entering, and the skills that your training isn't right now teaching you. Peter spent a decade trying to learn these skills; we offer them to you, right here in these pages. This book is your curriculum, to help you start off your career as a leader, a pioneer, and a doctor who not only won't need to be rescued himself, but who can rescue others.

Finally, if you're a policy maker, we want you to read this book to understand the challenges that often get swept aside in favor of broader debates about health care reform and improving the efficiency of health care delivery. Regulations and top-down mandates often fail because they're ignoring the people at the core of the system, whose needs must be central to any policy solution for it to have a chance at success: the doctors themselves. This book will give you the knowledge you need to better harness the skills and talents that doctors bring to the table, and to realize why so many current solutions are destined to fail.

We've spent years living in this world — on the doctor's side (Peter), and on the side of those who are tasked with coming in and working with doctors, to unleash their potential and use it to better the system for patients, administrators, policy makers, and the doctors themselves (Matt). Opening this book was the first step on your journey to rescuing the doctor. We hope to take you to the finish line, and give you the skills you need to transform not only your own professional lives but the entire health care industry.

* * *

> *"Research over the last few years has revealed that unrelenting job pressures cause two-thirds of fully trained doctors to experience the emotional, mental and physical exhaustion characteristic of burnout. Health care workers who are burned out are at higher risk for substance abuse, lying, cheating and even suicide. They tend to make more errors and*

lose their sense of empathy for others. And they are more prone to leave clinical practice."[2]

"A mentally healthy, highly motivated workforce might, in the short and long term, have greater impact on health care than a new drug."[3]

"I am a primary care doctor who started idealistic, and am disillusioned and dejected," wrote one reader from New York City: "By far, the biggest barrier to being a compassionate healer in our current working environment is time. We simply don't have the time we need to do our jobs well. And we all lose."[4]

"The husband of a doctor from Huntington, Pa., wrote that his wife, who worked 70 to 110 hours a week, was "constantly chafing against the demands for 'productivity,' the necessity to spend hours fighting insurers to get treatment for her patients and the fatigue that results from hours of work doing electronic 'paperwork' long after the patients have been seen."[5]

---

[2] http://well.blogs.nytimes.com/2013/09/26/easing-doctor-burnout-with-mindfulness/?_r=0

[3] JAMA Intern Med. 2013;173(8):709-710. http://archinte.jamanetwork.com/article.aspx?articleID=1681253.

[4] http://opinionator.blogs.nytimes.com/2013/10/02/who-will-heal-the-doctors/

[5] http://opinionator.blogs.nytimes.com/2013/10/02/who-will-heal-the-doctors/

"A survey of more than 13,000 doctors by the Physicians Foundation found that more than two-thirds of them feel negatively about their profession. Too much paperwork and regulations, plus the burden of defensive medicine, are the strongest contributors to this bleak outlook. These erode the doctor-patient relationship and the clinical autonomy that doctors have always cherished. What once seemed a higher calling increasingly feels like an assembly-line job."[6]

"In an online questionnaire of 24,000 doctors representing 25 specialties, only 54%, said they would choose medicine again as a career, down from 69% in 2011. Just 41% would choose the same specialty again. Only a quarter of doctors said they would choose the same practice setting, compared with 50% a year ago. Why such frustration and discontent among physicians? The Medscape survey cites declining incomes, excessive paperwork..."[7]

---

[6] http://ideas.time.com/2013/07/02/the-epidemic-of-disillusioned-doctors/

[7] http://www.forbes.com/sites/susanadams/2012/04/27/why-do-so-many-doctors-regret-their-job-choice/

REFRAME

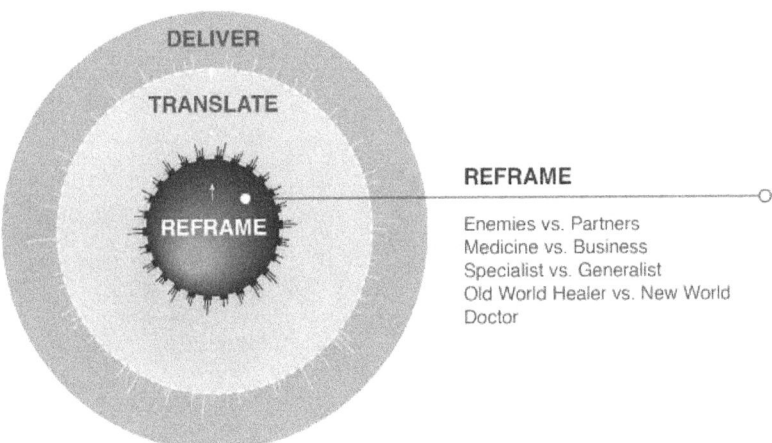

RESCUE THE DOCTOR

REFRAME

Enemies vs. Partners
Medicine vs. Business
Specialist vs. Generalist
Old World Healer vs. New World Doctor

THE DOCTOR'S DILEMMA: THE OLD WORLD IS BECOMING A NEW WORLD

A STORY

We're going to start with a story. The two of us have spent years talking to hundreds of doctors about their professional lives, their reasons for going into medicine, their biggest triumphs, and their greatest frustrations. So many doctors feel more pessimistic about their career choice than ever before. And that's putting it mildly — a recent study on burnout and satisfaction with work-life balance among U.S. physicians, published in the Archives of Internal Medicine, showed that nearly one in two doctors feels emotional exhaustion or in fact *regret* about their choice of career.[8]

---

[8] Arch Intern Med. 2012;172(18):1377-1385.

You may be one of those doctors, or you may work with dozens of those doctors. Or at least you may try to work with those doctors, but find them almost impossible to deal with. They're defensive, reactive, worried that the world of medicine is slipping from their grasp — or they're burned out, or checked out, unwilling to engage, unable to summon the motivation and drive they once had.

We talk to a lot of doctors who feel this way, but not a lot of doctors who understand *why* they feel this way. You can't even begin to address a problem that you don't fully comprehend. It's far too easy to accept these feelings of burnout and dissatisfaction as normal, unavoidable, and inevitable. It's hard to dig deeper and look for the reasons why — never mind figure out how to dig yourself out of the hole and get back on a fulfilling path.

What strikes us — over and over again — is how few doctors are seeing the big picture, understanding the drivers of change in health care and realizing that it's not just them as individuals who are feeling this way. Too often, doctors are blaming themselves — or blaming the people they work with and work for: "If only the hospital didn't have all of these rules...." "If only I had more control over my schedule...." "If only my patients weren't so demanding...." "If only they would give me more money to work with...." "...more people to work with...."

But none of these statements get at the much bigger picture, the huge changes that health care is undergoing around the globe, the forces affecting the industry at a level so much broader than in one particular hospital or even one particular country.

* * *

When we talk to doctors, and tell the story we're about to share, a light bulb turns on. Suddenly, they get it. Doctors are smart people — you wouldn't be a doctor if you weren't capable, intelligent, and ambitious. And the vast majority desperately want to do good, and have a deep sense of stewardship over their patients and over the world. But the more we've talked to doctors — and the more we've refined our story and made sure it reflects the reality of health care today — the more we've known we needed to write this book.

No one is providing doctors with the big picture and helping them understand that they're not alone, and that the frustrations they're feeling are not their fault. Reframing the current landscape — helping you to better see the world for what it is, recognize what is and isn't within your control, and increase your influence — is absolutely the first step toward rescuing yourself, your fellow doctors, and all of health care.

All of that said, our story starts with what we're calling the Old World. Medicine, for generations and generations, used to mean simply a doctor and a patient. From the time of Hippocrates, doctor were seen as high priests. They were respected and valued, and their decisions went unquestioned. Doctors were *lone healers*, relying on their clinical intuition above all, responsible to their patients and to themselves but ultimately to no one else.

We'll come back to this idea of *lone healers* a fair bit in the book — it's still so critical to how the world sees doctors and even how doctors see themselves, but, more and more, it is far removed from reality. And that disconnect is a huge part of the problem for a lot of doctors and how they feel about their profession.

Regardless of what the world looks like now, in the Old World things were far simpler. A good doctor recognized and diagnosed problems in his patients, built trusted relationships, and — a crucial piece — often worked entirely independently. Doctors were true independent knowledge workers, relied on not for speed and labor but for their intelligence and ability to inspect, observe, and analyze.

Doctors, in our story, could be thought of as the kings and queens of health care in the Old World, ruling over everything related to health and medicine. A doctor in the Old World works directly with his patients, of course. There's no clock to watch, no financial calculations to make, no meetings, no bureaucracy, no power struggles. His treatment decisions go unquestioned. There is no health care "system." There's him and his patients — that's all.

— This already does sound like an Old World, doesn't it? But this model lasted for centuries, in truth up until merely the last couple of generations. Medicine was always seen as different, and was always seen as driven entirely — entirely! — by the doctor. In the world of health care, the doctor wasn't only at the center of the model, he was truly the only player in the game. One of the most frustrating parts for doctors is that the Old World is still the world so many think they're entering — but who can blame them? It's the world they're being trained for!

There is one place left where it's only about the doctor and the patient — and that's medical school. Medical school, for the most part, strips away all of the external concerns — about business and finance, about dealing with administrators and colleagues, about internal and external politics — and, around the world, teaches future doctors as if the Old World were still in place. Doctors are not trained to run businesses or lead large, multidisciplinary teams — they're trained to heal patients. We'll discuss medical education in more detail later, but doctors can't be blamed for still seeing the world as it was for Hippocrates when it's all they've ever been taught. They're educated in the narrowest sense of what medicine is — still stuck in the old *lone healer* paradigm.

Over the past few decades, the Old World has started to shift. Health care isn't just about the doctor, and the doctor isn't the king. Or at least he isn't the only king. The core picture of medicine isn't that doctor-patient relationship anymore. In the New World, medicine is a technology park. It's a business center. It's filled with many diverse groups of people with competing interests and competing goals. The image on our cover is of imposing buildings staring down at that *lone healer*, of business and industry replacing the human touch.

Hippocrates didn't know hospital buildings; he knew one-on-one relationships. Now, medicine is about teams, not individuals. It's a shift away from just the doctor into the hands of doctors... plus an entire crew of other players, from administrators to policy makers to a finance team, legal, nurses and other patient care professionals, social workers, and so many more. If the Old World was a monarchy, and the doctor was king — well, in the new world, it's far more of a Parliamentary government.

— Before we get accused of going overboard: we're not saying doctors have been stripped of all their authority. Doctors are of course central to health care. The system can't exist without them, and even the most frustrated, jaded hospital bureaucrat would admit that he needs the doctor on the team. But that's our point: it's a *team* now, and doctors are just one of the players. They control some of our Parliamentary "seats," but other constituencies have a say as well. In the United States, there's the insurance companies. Across Europe, it's government. There are the drug companies, the people making medical equipment, policy makers, nurses, administrators, human resources, people setting the budget, lawyers... and the list goes on.

Doctors can't just make decisions unilaterally. Everything has to be discussed and justified. Coalitions have to be built. There are votes. There are trade-offs. And — here's the key — doctors don't always win. Sometimes they get overruled. They can't provide that treatment, or they can't offer that service, or they can't open that clinic, or they can't have that new machine, or they can't have funding for every project they want to undertake. Even if they're only thinking about the good of the patient. (Because, as most every doctor will insist, *of course* they're thinking about the good of the patient. Always. But resources are limited. In a way they simply never used to be.)

Doctors are not used to losing. But as medicine has gotten more complex, it has gotten more expensive. As it has gotten more expensive, there have to be limits. Not because any one player wants to put limits on what a doctor should be able to do, and what services should be provided, but because there is a finite amount of money in the system to allocate.

We've talked already about doctors getting burned out. This is much of the reason why. Having to fight for everything you want to do to help your patients is exhausting. Feeling like the ones who make the rules don't trust your clinical judgment — even if it's just a matter of budgets and choices — is exhausting. Especially without any training to know how a doctor in this New World needs to behave. New expectations placed on doctors to understand how the business of medicine operates, new demands that they follow rules and protocols, but often no training in these aspects of the job. Of course in response most doctors have the very understandable desire to bury their heads in the sand and hope it all goes away — hope the world stops changing and they can go back to just being doctors.

— Look, being a doctor was never easy. You could survey every doctor on the planet and none of them would say that they went into medicine because they wanted an effortless life. Long hours have always been a given, patients expect more than medicine can deliver, conditions are hard to diagnose, and treatments are never perfect. It's always been a purpose-driven career, a mission more than just a job.

But we talk to more and more doctors who say that something fundamental about the profession has changed. Doctors are struggling in ways they never have before. They're seeing themselves as victims in a workplace that has been taken over by administrators and bureaucrats looking for quick fixes, consultants bringing in the latest efficiency tools, forms and paperwork that have replaced time with patients, and a demand that they place economics above patient care. Their inability to meet these new expectations means that they're being pushed aside in their own industry, relegated to being mere employees instead of the ones making decisions and shaping their own professional lives — mere workers instead of men and women on a mission — driven by the clock instead of an inner compass.

These are new problems. In the Old World, doctors only needed to be concerned with the medicine; everything else would take care of itself. Not anymore. For every *lone healer* still seeing patients in his local office, practicing medicine the way it has been for a century, there are exponentially more doctors working within a larger, much more complicated system.

The trend is clear. The world isn't turning back. The Old World is becoming the New World, whether doctors like it or not. And that is the crux of the problem. The more doctors try to bury their heads in the sand and ignore the realities of the New World, the more the other players need to turn elsewhere for help. If doctors won't come on board, administrators are forced to try to engage nurses and others. They need doctors. They long for doctors to engage.

But if doctors won't engage, it doesn't mean the Old World system comes back. What it means is that doctors become more and more marginalized. It's a vicious cycle. Doctors disengage, managers turn to others, doctors become less crucial — then doctors get even more frustrated, and even more of them disengage. This is the doctor's dilemma that we refer to in the chapter heading.

* * *

So where are we in our story? Doctors thrived in the Old World, at the center of health care, but as medicine transitions to the New World, too many doctors are unable or unwilling to play along. Some fight against the inevitable, and some check out, going through the motions — and dragging others down with them — or literally leaving the profession. Others step in, gaining influence and power — and the health care world moves on without the doctor.

Sure, for a while, a doctor can cling to that Old World model and try to desperately hang onto that idea of the doctor-patient relationship being the only thing that matters. But the system is moving forward, and these doctors are stuck in the past. When everyone else has left for the New World, the Old World remains as a lonely island, drifting further away from the New World mainland.

Of course doctors are still needed on the mainland, in the big hospitals and complex medical systems that dominate the New World. Nurses can't do neurosurgery. The human resources department doesn't know how to allocate a doctor's budget most effectively for the patients. Managers are forced to reach out for the doctors' help — but if you think about that relationship, you start to realize it's the reverse of what it ought to be. Rather than doctors being the leaders, at the center of decision-making and using these other players to provide support and necessary administrative help, instead the doctors (having disengaged, and refusing to step up and lead) are on the margins, only consulted when absolutely necessary.

Managers are trying. They do want to engage doctors. But if doctors won't play ball, they're forced to make decisions themselves — not always the decisions the doctors would have made. Then, when the doctor is hit with a new set of rules, or told his clinic has to be closed, or given a slashed budget to work with — well, it only exacerbates the problem and drives everyone further and further apart.

And the Old World healers drift away. Further and further from the health care mainland where the important decisions are being made, further and further from the seats of power. And the more they distance themselves, the less important they become in the process, the less involved they become in running their own institutions, and the harder it becomes to ever find their way back.

— The doctors, as we've already said, will insist they're only looking out for the good of their patients. Choices like the ones they're being asked to make, they will argue, shouldn't be made at all. The problem, however, is that *the choices will be made*, either by them or by someone else. If they're allowing others to make those choices, then, ultimately, their patients are indeed being hurt despite their best intentions.

As time passes, the New World and what's left of the Old World grow further and further apart. Eventually, they're not even speaking the same language anymore. In the New World, they're speaking the language of business, of costs and benefits, checks and balances. The doctors don't understand — and aren't even trying to understand. They're not ready. They're just not prepared.

So the administrators are forced to work with as little input from the doctors as they can manage. Every time they try to reach out — throw a rope over to the Old World, try to pull some doctors across — they're met with skepticism and anger. They offer a training program, perhaps some new initiatives to help doctors bridge that gap — but the doctors see it as more top-down dictates from management, more uselessness that only serves to drive them further away. (Truth is, any traditional business and leadership training that management tries to introduce at this point is destined to fail — another reason we knew we had to write this book. It is just too soon for health care to embrace these initiatives. Even if you put aside the limitations of these programs, doctors aren't there yet. They don't understand the landscape —so it simply falls on deaf ears.)

— It is not the fault of the doctors. The rug has been pulled out from underneath them. They didn't ask for the world to change — it just did. They want to help. Doctors become doctors because they want to help people. But they don't have the skills that the New World requires. They don't have the ability — or, just as important, the *desire* — to think in terms of financial limitations and business trade-offs. They don't have the ability — or, again, the *desire* — to share power, to work together, to lead and manage, and to build teams.

Gaining these abilities is, in many ways, the easy part — and much of this book aims to help get doctors started. Having the desire to change is an entirely different issue, and it's one that no one has been addressing until now. But we hope to make the case that doctors can do more than just avoid burnout if they start to embrace the New World — they can in fact thrive and grow careers far more meaningful than the Old World was ever able to offer.

But we're getting ahead of ourselves. We still have more story to tell.

* * *

In the Old World, as more time passes, the burden on the doctors still fighting to remain in the past becomes greater and greater. More demands, more patients to see. Just like the New World needs doctors, doctors need the support that the New World can provide — for legal issues, for billing, for infrastructure, and more. But rather than working together, they're seeing their potential partners in the New World as enemies instead. It's a devastating way to look at your professional world, with you as the victim and everyone else fighting to take away your power. No wonder these Old World healers are getting burned out and even leaving the profession. It's hard to fight. It's discouraging. In the Old World, seeing the world move past you, it's easy to become disillusioned and forget why you became a doctor in the first place.

— A new, younger generation of doctors is witnessing the battle between the Old World and the New, sees the challenges and dysfunctions in the system, and, naturally, starts to question their choices before their careers even begin. What this means is that new doctors are less reluctant than ever to fully commit to medicine — and gravitating, more and more, to specialties that are merely shiftwork. They don't want the added responsibilities that the New World demands. They'll wring whatever benefits remain from the Old World and seek fulfillment elsewhere — in their families, hobbies, or side businesses. And, no, of course there's nothing wrong with a doctor seeking satisfaction in the other parts of his life, but it's a shame to give up the true reward that being a doctor has throughout history provided. Being a doctor has never been like other careers — it's always been more than a job, it's been a mission.

Until now.

The New York Times published a recent op-ed titled, "Who Will Heal The Doctors?" Readers wrote in about their struggles:

> *People who are caught in oppressive systems adopt various stances toward them, consciously or unconsciously. They may choose to abandon the systems; today many doctors are doing just that. Several wrote in to say that they had already quit medicine, or were planning to quit soon. 'I retired early from medicine, was glad to get out, and don't regret fleeing a broken system,' wrote J. Skinner from the Midwest."*[9]

Sadly, this is what being a doctor has come to. And the longer doctors try to stay on the Old World's lonely *Doctor Island*, the further it drifts from the New World and the future of medicine — and the more the profession is threatened. Even the most headstrong doctors cannot keep their heads buried in the sand forever. The current picture, unfortunately, is unsustainable.

The Old World will be washed away as doctors are hit with the perfect storm — a set of fundamental drivers powering New World medicine that are finally forcing change.

It has been a generation of struggle as the New World has drifted, leaving the Old World healers behind. But now, the Old World is being washed away.

---

[9] http://opinionator.blogs.nytimes.com/2013/10/02/who-will-heal-the-doctors/

This is why we're telling our story now. The forces outside of any doctor's control — which have contributed over recent decades to a dramatic shift moving doctors out from the center of the health care system — are finally coming to a head. The doctor is, of course, still a key player, and will always be a key player, but he is being buried by demands and realities that he can't quite dig his way out from underneath.

Peter started out, twenty years ago, like many doctors, motivated by all the right things, idealistic about the profession and the work he was set to devote his life to. But as he transitioned from being a pure clinician to a manager and leader of people, he realized that while he had the appropriate clinical training to serve his patients, that wasn't enough. He began a decade-long journey to fill in the gaps in his training. Working with Matt, who has spent his career helping hospitals try to get the most out of their doctors — and with doctors to try and get the most of their careers — we believe that together we have *cracked the code* for doctors to rescue themselves and, in turn, rescue the entire profession.

If you are an Old World healer, you are going to need to change how you view your role. That's simply the reality in today's world. You can't look at medicine the way it used to be and merely wish for everything to return to the way it was.

It isn't happening.

But this doesn't have to cause as much pain as you fear. Instead, it can create tremendous opportunity. Doctors who understand New World health care can regain their place at the center of the system, drive transformation, lead hugely satisfying and fulfilling careers, and be the real game-changers.

To get there, you need to understand what's driving the changes, and then you need to step back and take a look at yourself. You need to find your direction, develop a few critical skills, and take charge of your career.

If you embrace the change — if you commit to the challenge and do the necessary work — you can find a bridge back to the New World and rescue yourself, then your colleagues, and then your institution.

In the next section, we will delve deeply into these four key drivers of New World medicine — Enemies vs. Partners, Medicine vs. Business, Specialist vs. Generalist, and, finally, Old World Healer vs. New World Doctor.

Once you see health care through these New World eyes, you can begin your journey, recover what drove you to become a doctor, and once again find the joy that a career in medicine can bring.

For me, this journey is quite a personal one. Like so many doctors, I started out assuming that a passion for helping patients, combined of course with solid medical training, would be enough to sustain me no matter the twists and turns I would encounter in my career.

When I finished my medical training, I found myself one day writing a list — what I called my Life List, a set of great things I wanted to set my sights on and hope to achieve in my career. You may have done the same, if not on paper then at least in your mind. The things you're shooting for in the long run, the legacy you want to leave.

Of course, if you're reading this book you've already figured it out — great training and a passion for medicine aren't enough. Yes, you survive, and even thrive, but the longer I've been practicing medicine — and I suspect this holds just as true in so many different professions — I've realized that the people who end up with the most satisfying careers (and I don't necessarily mean the highest prestige or the highest pay — but the ones who seem truly fulfilled, happy, and productive) aren't necessarily the best trained, the ones with the most passion, or the ones who can best articulate their career goals.

As my career as a physician-scientist progressed, I saw, over and over again, what separated the true winners — those with the greatest impact and who left a real legacy — from everyone else had almost everything to do with character and other issues related to the human side of the equation.

When I say "character," I don't mean the image that people attempt to portray to the world, but I'm talking about something deeper than that, your true self — your personal integrity, your credibility, your trustworthiness, your ability to build positive and effective relationships, your purpose beyond just being out for yourself.

Figuring all of this out at first turned on its head everything I had valued most up until that point — my education, my skills, and my ambition. It was like seeing a 3D movie for the first time, when all I had known before was a flat, two-dimensional world: these human aspects, as never before, popped out from the background, and I realized that they were the critical (and for too long largely ignored) pieces in my professional life.

More and more, I shifted my focus from purely medicine and science to thinking about these issues of character and human interactions, and trying to fine-tune my skills in these areas. I did what doctors and scientists are trained to do and dove into the subject, looking for the magic answers.

I spent over a decade reading books much longer than this one, attending countless conferences, lectures, and workshops, and attempting to follow the wisdom of every guru out there. But it took me years to realize that I was searching for knowledge that didn't exist — no one was bringing these issues to health care and talking about them in a way that was relevant and useful to doctors and to our world.

Health care is getting more and more complex and in some ways leaving doctors behind. I absolutely believe it is these types of human issues that are standing in our way. I decided that I needed to tell my story, help doctors recognize the problems facing the profession and then learn (as I did) how to understand the changes and take the lead, returning doctors to the center of health care. I met Matt, and we began to work together on this book, and to bring Rescue The Doctor to the people who need it most.

Health care as an industry does not and cannot work without the doctors at the center. But to get back there, we all need to look at our careers in a new way, and embrace the changing role of the doctor rather than fighting it. My hope is that this book gets you on the path to rescuing yourself and others.

One doctor, with the right mindset, can indeed rescue himself. A handful of doctors can rescue a hospital. And, eventually, my hope is that many doctors can rescue the whole system, and truly lead medicine forward. We owe it to our patients, and to ourselves, to at least give it a try.

— Peter

THE DRIVERS OF NEW WORLD MEDICINE

The lesson took Peter years to learn: the problem isn't that doctors aren't working hard enough. That would be an easy answer, for sure, but it's wrong, and every doctor reading this book knows it's wrong. Indeed, much of the reason doctors are unhappier than at previous points in history is that they're working *too* hard — too many hours, too many demands, pulled in too many directions. And they think they only have to work harder. See more patients, see them faster, get more done — get ahead of the game, that's how to fix what's wrong.

It's not.

Working harder isn't the answer, working smarter is — but we'll get there. Truth is, the problems are bigger than any individual doctors — they're systemic. There are fundamental changes happening in the world, even outside of health care, that have changed the profession. We talk to doctors all the time who are, for lack of a better term, stuck in their own bubble. They aren't looking at the bigger picture. They think their problems are unique to them, their burdens, their frustrations, their dissatisfaction, their burnout, is *all about them*. But doctors are smart people — for years, we ended these conversations thinking, *if only doctors saw what was really happening, they could fix their problems on their own.* That's what started us on the road to writing this book.

Drifting into the core of new world medicine is an increased focus on profit, efficiency, and economics. Medicine used to be a safe haven from the pressures of business, but medicine also used to be a lot simpler, and a lot cheaper. There was less that doctors could do. But increased technology combined with breakthroughs in biomedical research have made possible precision medicine — new understanding at levels far more granular than a healer even just a few generations ago could have ever imagined.

Technology has enabled doctors to see and understand things they never before could. And it's obviously wonderful for patients and for the profession that we can do so much more than we used to, treating more illnesses, managing more conditions, extending life and restoring health. The problem is that someone has to pay for it. No matter the system, and no matter whether you're in the United States, Europe, or elsewhere, economics have become a huge concern. Doctors in previous generations did not have to worry much about the costs. Doctors today absolutely do.

Coupled with the economic pressures are a growing number of stakeholders in health care — in short, the people in charge of the money care how it's being used. So what used to be just doctors accountable to themselves is now doctors accountable to government, to politicians, to administrators at every level, to finance teams at their own institutions, and more. Doctors fear — often rightly, based on past experience — that health care is being taken over by people who don't know about medicine, who don't know about patients, and who don't have the patients' best interests at heart. At the same time, managers fear that doctors don't care about the bigger picture and just want to practice the way they always have, even when budgets weren't a concern. Neither side truly understands the other.

But the growing complexity of medicine isn't just affecting the cost of care and increasing the number of stakeholders — it's also affecting the way medicine has to be practiced. Doctors can't serve their patients as *lone healers* anymore — there is too much medicine for one person to understand. More and more, doctors are finding themselves in narrower and narrower specialties, and patients need to rely on an entire medical team — a team which, in an ideal world, would be interconnected and working as one. But the skills needed to work together with colleagues are much different than when you're on your own.

Related to all of this — and quite possibly the most devastating to a doctor's traditional feeling of satisfaction and fulfillment — is that the increased complexity of medicine and the growing reliance on technology have made doctors and their independent observation, thinking, and analysis vastly less integral to the job. Doctors have, in many ways, gone from being independent knowledge-age workers to dependent industrial-age workers, functioning in a world of assembly-line medicine.

It's not a small thing at all, as far as what the day-to-day practice now looks like. The doctor's job itself is far more routinized than ever before — he's seeing a narrower and narrower band of patients, focusing his practice around a smaller number of issues and treatments, following a script instead of needing to use a broader range of skills and intuition.

The economic factors along with the technology have made this unavoidable. A doctor can see ten times the number of patients with an EKG than a stethoscope. A doctor can earn a hospital ten times more money spending his day doing procedures rather than talking to patients. The economic incentives, sadly, don't match the kind of work doctors have traditionally valued.

And there's a larger point to be made here. At the same time as tools are replacing brains for doctors, others in the medical field — most notably, nurses — have seen themselves on the reverse journey, rising from industrial-age assembly line workers to knowledge workers, empowered to do more than ever before. We'll go into more detail later, but nurses are now managing people and managing patients, providing much of the hands-on care that used to give doctors much of their sense of worth in the workplace.

It's been too easy for an individual doctor to close his eyes and hope these shifts would simply go away, or not affect him. Most doctors went into medicine to treat patients — so that's what they've kept on doing. Treating patients, more and more of them, faster and faster. With no time to look over their shoulders and see the impending storm approaching.

We've identified a set of four drivers that encompass these shifts in health care and that are powering New World medicine. In the pages that follow, we'll dive deeper into each. Together, they explain what we see as happening in the world, and what doctors must understand before they can rescue themselves. Without fully understanding the shifting ground on which they stand, doctors can't take control, and can't begin their journey back to satisfaction, medical leadership, and fulfilling careers.

Enemies vs. Partners

The new stakeholders in medicine — management, finance, politicians, lobbyists and regulators, lawyers, nurses, more educated patients, medical technology firms and device manufacturers — are seen by many doctors, far too often, as threats. Threats to their independence, threats to their authority, threats to their power and prestige, and, most critically, threats to the care they want to provide and feel is best for their patients. But these feelings come too frequently from fear and lack of understanding the perspectives of these new influencers than from reality. Seeing them as enemies is stressful, counterproductive, and, frankly, incorrect. They're partners, and doctors not only have to work with them, but can get a lot more accomplished if they learn to do so effectively.

Medicine vs. Business

Modern medicine is, for better or worse, a big business — and doctors need to understand it as such. The *lone healer* model is no longer the rule, and just seeing patients is no longer enough. Doctors need to create room in their minds (and in their schedules!) for new activities — planning, strategy, budgeting — that they have traditionally been insulated from, not to mention never trained to do. Ignoring the realities of business, as tempting as that might be, will not make these issues go away. And only by understanding what the business side of medicine means and what the business stakeholders are looking for can doctors thrive in this new model.

Specialist vs. Generalist

Doctors have been trained to think as specialists. That means diving deep and becoming an expert. Peter's journey is perfect evidence — for a decade, he tried to learn everything he could about business and become an expert, like he would if a new disease or condition emerged that he needed to be able to treat. He was thinking like a doctor. But all of that thinking led nowhere, and took away from his core purpose as a clinician. Doctors in the New World need to think like generalists when it comes to the issues beyond clinical ones — they need to have enough of an understanding to engage and know how the pieces fit together, but they don't need to be the experts in everything, and certainly don't need to try to solve every problem themselves. They need to rely on the experts around them — which is something doctors are not necessarily used to doing.

Old World Healer vs. New World Doctor

What makes a good doctor has changed. No longer is it just diagnosis and treatment that makes a doctor successful, happy, and valued. Those are merely the cost of entry — it's assumed that you're a good clinician. The question is whether you're a team player, an asset to the whole organization, and a partner not only with your patients but with all of your new stakeholders. A New World doctor needs more skills than the Old World healers were historically expected to have, and professional success in the health care world is simply not just about clinical expertise. Ignoring this reality — as so many doctors unintentionally end up doing — only creates frustration, missed opportunities for career growth, and, ultimately, the burnout we're trying to avoid.

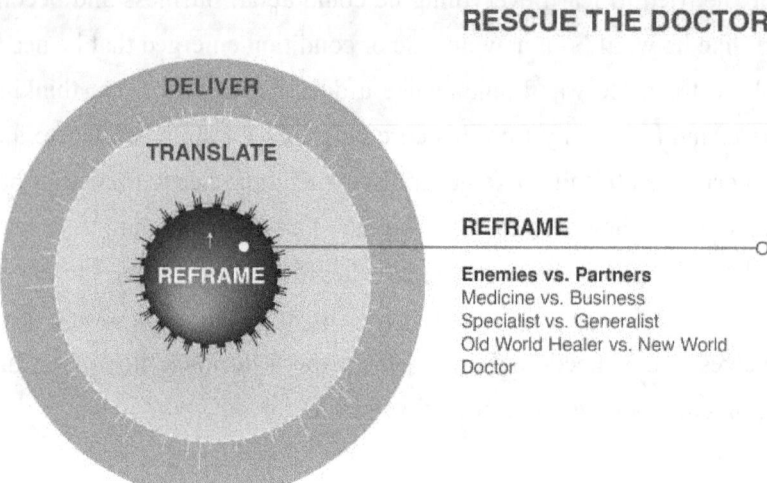

ENEMIES VS. PARTNERS

No one would blame doctors for feeling like victims. For generations they were not just in charge, they were everything. Unquestioned, unchallenged, independent. Now, everyone is coming at them with new rules, limitations, and demands. Managers are telling them what to do — or at least it feels like they are. Finance is making patient care decisions — or at least it feels like they are. Politics is affecting their workplace — what services their hospital can provide, or even whether their hospital can stay open. Nurses are becoming more influential. Patients — more informed than ever before — are showing up with Internet printouts and demanding certain care.

Technology is replacing the thinking that used to be the doctor's core competency. Freedom and autonomy feel very much threatened. Doctors feel backed into a corner, made to see more and more patients, faster and faster, with fewer resources, more meetings, directives, regulations, and paperwork, fewer financial rewards despite longer hours, more headaches, more bureaucracy, more of everything except the kinds of things they became a doctor in order to do, like talking to patients, feeling like they're helping people, feeling like they're making a difference.

It never used to be this way, they think, and while in some ways they're surely romanticizing the past, in many ways they aren't. It is not their imagination, even if they're made to feel that way by administrators who don't understand why the doctors aren't cooperating and being "team players." Things really have changed, and it's awfully easy for a doctor to say they've changed for the worse. Everyone wants something from them. No one will leave them alone. They're being coerced into following new efficiency protocols — or at least that's how it feels. And it doesn't seem to benefit the patients — or at least that's how it feels.

If you're reading this and you're not a doctor, you need to realize this: doctors feel like victims, even if it's not your intention to make them feel that way. Doctors see their independence evaporating — and they're not wrong. The world really is different.

As human beings, our natural reaction to a situation like this is to demonize the people making often-unrealistic demands of us — or at least demands we don't quite agree with — and turn them into the enemy. What do you do when threatened by an enemy? You either back down and submit — accept defeat, and either become a burnout statistic or leave the profession entirely — or you stand up and fight back. You refuse to play the game. You stand up to management and stand up to finance, and you keep on doing things the way you've always done them. You skip meetings — or you text your way through them. You promise to be a team player and then do the minimum you possibly can. You grumble and snort and have absolute conviction that you're in the right because you're doing it all for your patients. You're standing up for yourself so that you can devote yourself to patient care. How dare they expect you to spend your energy defending your turf and fighting administrators when you should be taking care of your patients? How dare they put their needs ahead of your patients? If only they would leave you alone....

* * *

Have we made a compelling case here? Are doctors the victims? You can certainly understand why it's easy for them to see it that way. And we're not going to tell doctors they aren't victims. It's naïve to pretend that some of the changes to health care haven't made life more difficult for them. It's absurd to pretend that doctors should be on board with everything that's changed about the profession. But here's what we tell doctors who insist that they're victims and that everyone around them is the enemy:

IT DOESN'T MATTER.

Whether you want to call yourself a victim or not, it's irrelevant, because the reality is that these stakeholders do have a voice. And so, as a doctor, you have a choice. You can fight — and lose. Or you can change your mindset and figure out how to work with these other functions — and partner with them for the good of your patients and the good of your own professional growth and satisfaction. As naïve as it is to pretend that doctors aren't affected by the New World of medicine, it's just as naïve to pretend that anyone who's not a doctor is out to get doctors, and wants to hurt patients. They don't — or at least there's no reason to ever assume they do.

What too many doctors don't stop to realize is that management has demands placed on them just like they're seeing demands placed on themselves. Budgets are limited. Resources are scarce. And for doctors to continue doing the work they do, they need management to figure out ways to make the economics work. They need management to do the work they do so that doctors don't have to do it themselves, and can keep spending their time on patient care. Management sees themselves as helping doctors the best they can, and they usually are. So, to them, doctors are the ones who are the enemies — fighting change, fighting reason, and fighting the reality of what has to happen in order for health care to survive.

Choices need to be made. Doctors don't want to make them. Entirely understandable, but they still have to be made. So the doctors run away, and treat the ones who do end up making hard choices as enemies — and instead of good solutions and cooperation, we end up with a dysfunctional, fragmented system where everyone is fighting with one another.

* * *

When you look at everyone around you as an enemy, you take on a defensive posture. You interpret everything as an attack, even if it's not intended to be. You see the worst in each other, and you expect the worst to come. New directives from management are pounced on and attacked, without being given a fair look. In turn, questions from doctors are seen as accusations, and aren't given legitimate consideration. Does the fighting make anyone happy? Of course not. We know from the burnout study that the current situation isn't satisfying anyone.

What's desperately needed is a change in how doctors — and those working with doctors — see the world. It's not an easy change. It would be relatively simple to just say to both sides: *stop fighting*. Placate each other. Put your heads down and get back to work, disengage, ignore the attacks. But disengaging can't possibly be the goal. Disengaging doesn't help — the patients, or the doctors. Fighting's bad, sure. But you can't replace fighting with avoidance.

Along the same lines, it would be easy to say to doctors: *yes, you're right*. You do know what's best for your patients, and these other people are only getting in your way. Your efforts to stand up to them aren't working, not because you're not justified but because you're not committed enough. Everyone is in fact your enemy, stealing your power and authority, and the answer is to start a doctor revolution. Wait, no — this deserves capital letters — A Doctor Revolution. Hit them where it hurts. There can't be health care without doctors, so you have all of the leverage. Don't back down. Fight for every dollar, fight back against every directive, attack every decision. You will win — maybe not all of the time, but some of the time. And isn't winning the goal? (Hint: the answer is no.)

Where would that leave us? It's still a war, whether you're winning or you're losing. In reality, there is no winning or losing, because if you "win," health care becomes unaffordable, or untenable in the political climate.

Management needs doctors, and doctors — perhaps reluctantly — do need management or they won't be able to keep practicing medicine. But it's not about reluctantly putting down your guns and calling a truce. It's not about capitulating to the demands of others. For the sake of the patients and for the sake of the system, it has to be about *changing your paradigm*. It has to be about coming together to find answers that are better than managers can come up with alone, without the help of doctors — and answers that are also better than doctors can come up with alone, without an understanding of the bigger picture and the concerns of all the stakeholders who have a say in the system.

It's about partnership. Because as hard as it sometimes is to see it, everyone is actually on the same side. Ideally, they're all fighting for the patients, just with different tools. Doctors have their clinical tools, but finance has tools as well, as do politicians and nurses and everyone else in the system. No one is setting out to hurt doctors — and, doctors, you have to realize that. They're just trying to manage a system that is bigger than you, and that you can't ignore. Circumstances are real. Budgets are finite. Time is finite. You have no choice but to work together if you want to succeed.

As difficult as you find it to deal with the bureaucracy, they find it just as difficult to deal with doctors. Matt's experience bears this out — and we'll absolutely cover this in more detail later: management is desperate to engage doctors, they just don't know how. Everyone's on a different island, to use the metaphor from our story earlier, and speaking different languages. That has to change.

There's a perception that health care is a see-saw. One group gaining influence means that someone else is losing it. But that's not true, any more than it's true that one patient getting better means another must be getting worse. Partnership is a good thing for doctors, a good thing for health care, and a good thing, ultimately, for patients.

We can break the doctor's world down, group by group. How doctors see each set of stakeholders, how they see doctors, what's really going on, and how to move forward. By peeling back the layers of suspicion and mistrust that have driven all sides to their corners, we can get to a clean slate, and help everyone realize it doesn't have to be a battle. If we can move from enemies to partners, and understand this first driver powering the New World of health care, we can then finally begin to rescue the profession.

Doctors vs. Management

> *"Physicians often feel that the solutions to their issues are clear cut and may become impatient with the time it takes to hear from multiple voices before making a decision. Administrators become frustrated when, in the interest of expediency, the physician moves forward before discussing the impact on the rest of the organization or raises concerns after decisions have been carefully made. The differences might be*

> *summed as follows: Physicians tend to focus on the individual; hospital administrators tend to focus on the enterprise."*[10]

> *"Doctors and managers have different cultures, which opens up possibilities not only of fruitless fighting but also of rich learning."*[11]

This section is the largest because, to doctors, management is the primary enemy in this New World of health care — although by no means the only one. See, to many doctors, the mere existence of managers, outside of their own ranks, is itself a threat. Historically, doctors *were* the leaders: *they themselves were management.* Health care was run by doctors, and exclusively by doctors.

Of course, that was a world of solo practitioners and *lone healers*, not the hospital-based system that the health care industry has become. Clearly a management layer of some sort is necessary to run these large health care organizations — doctors have neither the time nor, in most cases, the skills that managers are supposedly bringing to the table. But even if doctors would have to admit that management is necessary, it is still a huge change for them to go from positions of leadership to a subservient position where they are merely the employees, like the workers on a factory line.

In the eyes of the Old World healer, the introduction of a management layer — outsiders brought in to run medical organizations — is where things first started to derail. It meant a change from a profession built on character to one that was forced to focus on efficiency over everything else. Medicine became about processes, budgets, and an assembly line mentality, not about

---

[10] http://www.healthcarestrategygroup.com/newsletters/article.php?show=engaging_physicians_why_the_tensions_part_2_

[11] http://www.ncbi.nlm.nih.gov/pmc/articles/PMC1125519/pdf/610.pdf

knowledge and thought — and doctors went from leaders to servants. Instead of a craft, medicine became a factory job. And burnout has naturally followed.

From the doctor's perspective, these managers — who in most cases have no clinical training — are trying to influence the treatment of their patients. That naturally makes doctors very uncomfortable. The more mandates, rules, standards, and dictates that come down from management — the more paperwork, meetings, demands, and requirements — the more doctors chafe at the interference. This is the root of their unhappiness. To them — many of them — it feels like their industry is being stolen out from under them, and their wisdom has been replaced by bean-counting and number-crunching.

Of course that's not the only way to look at things. Managers would argue that their existence is allowing doctors to keep practicing medicine instead of having to run businesses — something they aren't trained to do anyway. And managers would insist that they're absolutely not looking to dictate how doctors practice medicine, or looking to steal power. They want doctors to be as involved as they're willing to be as far as setting policy and making the rules — but the problem is that doctors are unwilling to step up. Managers would say that they're doing everything they can to protect the doctor — but that doctors are unwilling to accept the reality that there are limitations, in terms of time and money. And that there is good to be gained from standardization, reporting, and accountability — things that doctors have notoriously been bad at throughout history.

Management needs the cooperation and involvement of doctors to develop and validate new processes, and to implement new ideas. They desperately want to bring doctors on board. But the doctors are stuck in their Old World view, managers would argue. They won't support anything that management wants to do, they're not willing to listen, and eventually management has no choice but to stop wishing for cooperation and force doctors to do things their way.

This, of course, plays into the doctor's fears that management is trying to steamroll over them, bad feelings continue, doctors see themselves as the victim, and we end up where we are today. Plans don't get implemented, efforts fail, and, in the end, you don't get safer surgery or the optimal allocation of resources... and patients get hurt.

There is truth on both sides of the divide. Health care has become too big of a business for doctors to run it themselves, or at least for doctors to run it and still practice medicine. There are studies that show great advantage for hospitals to be run by doctors, but finding doctors with the business skills — and, more importantly, the interest — to give up their white coats and become management is challenging. And when they do switch sides, their colleagues are likely to see them as doctors no longer, and feel the same sense of mistrust they do when it's outsiders leading the organization.

But managers are not completely innocent either. They often chase the wrong priorities and the wrong initiatives, inviting doctors to be skeptical of their intentions. They bring generic business tools to health care when health care truly is different — and managers lose their credibility in the process. Finally, managers say they want doctors to be involved but too often they don't act as if that's true, and doctors have legitimate reasons to worry.

The answer here is the same as the answer is going to be for all of the different stakeholders. Both sides are stuck with each other, and no amount of screaming or wishing is going to turn back the clock or change the reality. So there's a choice to make: do you continue fighting, to the detriment of your patients and yourselves, or do you recognize the reasons for the tension, and then find a way to get on the same page, chase the common goal of improving patient care, and work together as partners?

In a book chapter on mending the gap between doctors and hospital executives, J. Deane Waldman and Kenneth H. Cohn write:

"The common values and concerns shared by physicians and healthcare executives could provide the framework for successful communication leading to a bridge across the gap and a collaborative rather than confrontational relationship. Physicians could teach healthcare executives about clinical priorities, useful new technologies, and scientific methodology, including evidence-based decision making. Healthcare executives could educate physicians about management tools and techniques for planning, implementation, and assessment, especially systems thinking. Together as partners, healthcare executives and physicians could address many of the currently insoluble problems in healthcare."[12]

That, in the end, is what a rescued system should look like, in terms of doctors and managers. That, in the end, is New World medicine.

Doctors vs. Finance

Separate from management specifically are the finance professionals, seen as particular enemies by Old World healers who are used to unlimited budgets and unquestioned care. To doctors, seeing finance as the enemy is easy — they're telling doctors they can't do the things they want to do to serve their patients, whether it's buying a new piece of equipment, hiring a new secretary, adding additional staff, or bringing more doctors to the team. Doctors simply aren't used to monetary considerations infiltrating into patient care — and they feel like they have the moral high ground in saying that these financial factors shouldn't trump patient care. So it's obvious why

---

12

http://healthcarecollaboration.typepad.com/healthcare_collaboration_/files/physhosp gap_waldman.pdf they would have particular scorn for the people refusing to grant them unlimited access to the bank account.

What doctors tend not to think about is how difficult they make the job of the finance professional. In business, everyone is trained from day one to pay attention to the budget, but in medicine it's simply not how doctors are taught to think. So doctors, by and large, have absolutely no idea how they spend money. In training — and this is just about as close to a universal as these things get — doctors are deliberately kept in the dark about how much things cost, and how the economics of a hospital really work. So it's no surprise that when they get into practice, it just isn't something they think about. It's not seen as relevant to their job — which is to provide patients the best treatment they can, regardless of cost — so they ignore it.

Ignoring the money translates to the finance team as doctors being unable to stick to budgets, unwilling to accept budgets, and impossible to work with. And, in many cases, they are. Doctors will claim that patient care trumps everything — and then there is no argument left for finance to make. Doctors won't always accept that a dollar spent in one place means that there is one dollar less for everything else.

Believe it or not — and most doctors don't — finance wants doctors to succeed. They just need them to understand the limits. If you start with the premise that doctors and finance are on the same team, they don't have to be enemies. Instead, doctors get entrenched in their view that finance is trying to stop them from effectively treating patients. And it's a very short road from there to all-out war.

Doctors vs. Politics

It's the outsider problem here again, just as with managers: people without clinical knowledge trying to control the way medicine is practiced. Doctors see politicians as enemies because they're trying to influence medicine from the outside, with their own agendas (that don't always match up to the doctor's agenda). A good doctor isn't making decisions based on the optics — how things look to the public. He's trying to serve his patients, and no one else. That isn't how politics works.

At the same time, politicians are frustrated for the same reasons as managers are — the doctors won't engage. To politicians, doctors come off as arrogant, above the fray, unwilling to yield even an inch and help themselves by making it easier for politicians to advocate for them. They're seen as unwilling to change — and, largely, they are.

Again, the answer, to some extent, is easy. Politics exists. Decisions aren't made in a vacuum and some of the considerations are going to based in something other than the medicine itself. The hospital that is going to have to close is not always going to be the ones the doctors would choose. That doesn't change the fact that doctors can help themselves by engaging and not simply trying to pretend that they don't need to.

Doctors vs. Nurses

In some ways, this is a different problem than the others we've listed here so far. Nurses have been part of the system for far longer than managers or finance, and doctors have relied on them to help care for patients. The issue now is which side the nurses are on — management, or the doctors'? As doctors have disengaged and become more and more difficult for management to work with, in many cases management has turned to nurses to fill the gaps. Nurses are cheaper, and don't historically carry the same expectations that doctors do, as far as being in complete charge. Nurses are used to working as part of a team. For doctors, that's sometimes a bit more of a challenge.

The growing professionalism of nurses — the rise of roles like nurse practitioner and nursing manager — is evidence of a trend. As doctors fall in prestige and lose clout, on their journey from knowledge workers to assembly-line technicians, nurses are on their way up, moving into offices, taking on new roles, and asked to use their minds beyond just performing the manual labor we often associate with them. Of course it's good for patients to have more engaged and educated nurses. And of course the health care world is big enough for nurses to take on new roles without infringing on the job of the doctor. But not every doctor sees it that way.

The specialization of doctors means that nurses have become the ones providing much of the front-line patient care. Indeed, the rise of nurse practitioners and physician assistants has blurred the line between doctors and nurses. In the United States in particular, lower-paid medical specialties, like primary care, have seen a doctor shortage, and nurses have been deployed to fill in those gaps — cost-effectively and, in the eyes of many, without significant disadvantages. Forbes Magazine writes, "there are lots of losers in President Obama's effort to remake the U.S. health care system, and chief among them are the doctors. But there are also winners, especially nurses and physician assistants (PAs). Indeed, nurses and PAs win big in part because doctors lose badly."[13]

As doctors disengage more and more — entrenched in their Old World beliefs — there is room for nurses to take on responsibility. It is tempting for doctors to see nurses as stealing roles they used to have, and competing for the limited resources now available — doctors fighting with the head of nursing for resources and budget, for instance, when that never used to be the case.

Seeing nurses as competition for resources is not useful for doctors or for patients. Doctors need nurses — to provide the hands-on care that doctors don't have the time nor the skills to — and nurses need doctors as well. More than any of the other relationships in this section, the need for these groups to be partners in order to best care for patients is obvious, and the enemy mentality is clearly a destructive one.

---

[13] http://www.forbes.com/sites/merrillmatthews/2011/12/21/health-care-future-bright-for-nurses-stinks-for-doctors/

Doctors vs. Informed Patients

With the rise of the Internet, patients have more access to information, research, and each other. Doctors are reviewed by patients online. Patients bring stacks of printouts for doctors to respond to, and feel empowered to push back when a doctor gives them less time, or less attention. It's not the way the relationship used to be. Doctors were kings — unchallenged, undoubted. And, on the other side, patients were the doctor's entire world — but now there are other concerns — business concerns — on every doctor's plate.

Doctors worry that patients want and expect too much. Too many patients don't respect that a New World doctor isn't on call 24/7, and can't spend an hour with them — indeed, management and finance won't let them. They blame the doctor for the twenty-minute slots he's forced to subdivide his day into, and they blame him that medicine has gotten too complicated for one doctor to know everything, solve all of their problems, and see them on a moment's notice.

These are the reasons patients see doctors as the enemy. Doctors are hard to get hold of, and don't have the time. Obviously, new expectations need to be set, on both sides. There is no choice but for them to find a way to be partners and work together.

The other piece of this struggle between doctors and patients is the legal system. The threat of lawsuits hangs over every doctor's head in today's world, coming with it the skyrocketing cost of liability insurance and the huge number of hours doctors spend over the course of their careers devoted to handling malpractice claims — an estimated four years for the average doctor spent involved in active lawsuits — "more time than they spent in medical school," according to a study published in *Health Affairs* and covered by Pauline Chen of *The New York Times*.[14]

---

[14] http://well.blogs.nytimes.com/2013/01/24/the-drawn-out-process-of-the-medical-lawsuit/

The practice of defensive medicine — ordering more tests and procedures than medically necessary, in the hope of avoiding lawsuits — eats up a doctor's time and energy, and litigation-minded patients have become an enemy because of the mountains of paperwork they now force doctors to handle. Aggressive advertising by lawyers has planted ideas in patients' heads that doctors are the enemy, and it has made patients that much more ready to sue.

Doctors vs. Technology

This last battle is less about stakeholders and more about the changing role — and changing value — of a doctor. There is a temptation for doctors to see technology as an enemy because it has enabled people, for the first time in the history of medicine, to truly question the value of a doctor. Is a doctor really necessary when a machine can do the work at a fraction of the cost? Or when others — nurses and technicians — can do 90% of the work for 20% of the cost? FORTUNE magazine writes that computers will soon replace 80% of what doctors do. "Much of what physicians do," the magazine writes, "can be done better by sensors, passive and active data collection, and analytics... even [diagnosing and treating] better than the average doctor (while considering more options and making fewer errors)."[15]

Yes, doctors are still critical — especially if they can embrace a broader set of roles and responsibilities, and lead the people around them. But, with technology as advanced as it is, they are no longer the beginning and the end of medicine. Which is why the technology is so frightening. Patients still want to see the doctor, not the machine — for now. But it's not a given that won't change. So it's just one more in our long list of relationships the doctor needs to rethink and reconsider.

---

[15] http://tech.fortune.cnn.com/2012/12/04/technology-doctors-khosla/

We know we haven't provided any answers yet. These opposing constituencies are real, and destructive in a world where everyone is seen as an enemy. Finding a way to work together with all of these stakeholders — as partners — is key to rescuing doctors, and rescuing the system. But enemies vs. partners is only one of the drivers of new world medicine. Taken together with the three to come, we're hoping in this *reframe* section of the book to paint a picture of the current situation, and explain what's going on. In the sections ahead, we'll provide some skills to *translate* these ideas into practice and *deliver* breakthrough results — but for now, we think it's critical that doctors and others are aware of the landscape.

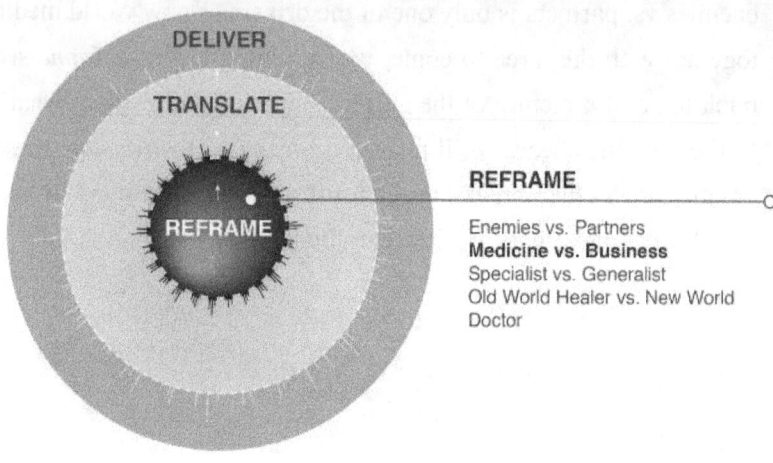

MEDICINE VS. BUSINESS

In almost any other industry, workers have traditionally had far more exposure to the concerns of business than doctors have in medicine — especially doctors who work in a hospital setting, where they aren't responsible for paying their staff directly, or for their office infrastructure. Even doctors who own their own practices are still insulated from many of the sales and marketing concerns that affect virtually every other profession. Yes, some doctors do market themselves, and even advertise — but many if not most doctors make few attempts to recruit patients, certainly not spending money to do so, and still they find themselves with greater patient loads than they can handle. The ones that do actively solicit patients are likely risking some loss of respect among their colleagues — at least their Old World colleagues who may see these types of activities as unseemly or beneath the dignity of the profession. It is a double-edged sword in some ways that doctors have historically been held to a higher standard than others. On one hand they are largely excused from thinking about business concerns — but on the other hand, they've never been able to develop those skills or taught to understand that world.

In terms of larger economic issues, health care, more than any other field, has few of the standard supply and demand concerns. No matter the overall economic health of a society, people will get sick, and doctors will be needed. Most critically, at the level of individual patients and individual treatment decisions, doctors are trained — and expected, if not by everyone, then at least by most of their patients — to ignore the cost of diagnosis and treatment when making patient care decisions and simply try to practice the best medicine that current knowledge and technology allow.

But while ignoring costs can certainly be justified when it comes to making choices for an individual patient (especially one whose only hope for recovery lies with an expensive treatment), when spread out over the entire system, the model has become less and less sustainable. In the past, medicine was simpler and cheaper — health care was not going to bankrupt a nation. But now, there really is a limited pool of money to go around, and — somewhere in the system — choices have to be made. The question for doctors isn't whether business concerns are going to have an effect on medicine — because they are — but whether these concerns are going to be addressed with the help of doctors, bringing their clinical wisdom to the table, or over in the halls of government, in the CEO suites, and in the number crunchers' offices down the hall, without doctor input and quite possibly with less-than-optimal results.

The fundamental problem as medicine moves from the Old World to the New is that most doctors simply do not accept that there is a limited budget, and that if the hospital doesn't make money, the patients will lose. According to one survey, only 36% of doctors see cutting costs as their responsibility.[16] That leaves 64% still stuck in a mindset that no longer reflects reality. It is absolutely true that for a long time, hospitals didn't have to worry about profits and doctors didn't have to concern themselves with costs. Health has always been seen as a special issue, and the money spent on it has been seen as more important than money spent elsewhere. Business is about making money; health care is about doing good. When there was enough money to go around, it was fine to let doctors run the show. But that was before hospitals were evaluated on a money-making basis, before the added scrutiny happening today, the increased analysis and limitations. Not to mention the widespread information now available.

Truth is, the public was in the dark for a very long time when it came to the business of medicine — and, indeed, the medicine of medicine, knowing which doctors and hospitals had the best outcomes, the most experience, and the fewest complications. Information now is everywhere. Data is much more easily collected and shared. Salaries are often public. Costs and results can be compared across doctors, across hospitals, and across countries. This has led — for the first time in history — to a chance for real accountability. In the past, even if someone wanted to hold doctors and hospitals accountable for their behavior and their expenditures, the data wasn't there. Now, we have enough information to power analysis and judgment. And so doctors need to justify their actions more than ever before. (In that same spirit, doctors also need to rely on their colleagues in a way

---

[16] http://healthpopuli.com/2013/07/24/doctors-not-keen-to-put-their-own-skin-in-the-u-s-health-care-cost-game/

they never did. It used to be that a good doctor was only judged on his own merits, but now a good doctor can be affected by bad data from his hospital.)

Increasingly, attempts are being made to standardize care — within an institution, and across institutions. Part of this is driven by outcomes, and wanting to make sure that best practices are followed everywhere. Part of it, inevitably, is driven by costs. Doctors are now facing limits on the treatments they can provide, or the equipment they can use. There is scrutiny and analysis where before there was freedom. And that, in some ways, gets at the core of the issue for doctors. Before business concerns reared their head in medicine, there was freedom. But business has brought with it restrictions and limitations — a loss of freedom — and doctors blame business instead of blaming the realities of a limited budget.

* * *

Doctors can no longer merely hope these changes go away. They need to become savvy about business, enough to understand the financial model of their institutions and how decisions get made. They don't need to become experts — and we'll discuss this further as we talk about the Specialist vs. Generalist driver — but they do need to be informed enough to become involved in the choices, rather than letting others take over that process completely.

That is the fundamental struggle here — doctors are losing because, without realizing it, they have opted out of the business decisions, but failed to realize those decisions still must be made. The decisions are thus made by others, without the same clinical knowledge and care that the doctors have — so, of course, once the decisions are made, the doctors disagree, and fight. Those making the decisions end up being treated as enemies, doctors withdraw further into their own silos, and the downward spiral continues. Business and medicine end up at war with each other instead of working together for the good of the patients.

But it's not just about business training.

If it were, this would be easy. We would tell doctors everything they need to know about business, wrapped up in a simple course, and everyone would live together in perfect harmony. This is the trap Peter fell into when he spent a decade trying to become a business expert.

It is not about doctors becoming business experts, because doctors are already busy enough being medical experts and treating patients.

And it is definitely not about introducing business training into a world that has shown no sign of a willingness to accept it. Even if business training would ultimately help doctors, we're three steps behind right now. We're not even at the point that most doctors will admit that costs matter to them, let alone ready to actually address those costs.

Which is why business training efforts up to this point have failed — and often dramatically so. It is far too easy for business to think it can come in and solve medicine, for outsiders to step in as the heads of hospitals and say they can fix things. They see medicine like a production line, and so they think they can introduce tools that have worked elsewhere, and — without an understanding of what makes medicine different — expect results.

There have been times we have started to explain Rescue The Doctor to an audience, and the quick response is for a doctor to sigh and ask why they need yet another business training tool — when they're already bombarded all the time with new management training courses, and administrators bringing in the latest and greatest efficiency tools (none of which have a chance of working because doctors won't accept them).

Hospitals have tried to implement general business training systems like Lean and Six Sigma with little to show for it. The Kings Fund in the UK, for instance, looked at Lean and concluded:

> *"The culture change that Lean demands is based on efficiencies in the the flow of production. It fails to include the human values that are essential in a high stress, high turnover environment of*

*hospitals where the outcome has to be measured in clinical and personal as well as financial terms."*17

Sure, efficiency is a problem in medicine — waste can certainly be cut from the system — and of course there are specific efficiency tools that could make a difference. But it's not just about throwing efficiency tools at hospitals and seeing what sticks. Medicine isn't just about efficiency: doing things quickly doesn't matter if you're doing the wrong things. Sick people aren't interchangeable like widgets. They're all different, not all of them will have good outcomes no matter the quality of the care provided, and each patient visit can quite legitimately take a different amount of time. You can't measure patients like you can measure parts on an assembly line, and you can't apply one-size-fits-all algorithms to treating patients.

Medicine, doctors will insist, and insist correctly, is far more complex. Each problem is genuinely different and each patient has a genuinely different combination of medical issues to consider. Before business factors even come into play, the medical decision making is complicated enough. To add more complexity to a complex world is naturally overwhelming to the doctor. Business outsiders don't always recognize this unique complexity — and the unique stakes that medical treatment has for its customers, in a way that almost any other service provided does not.

Instead, business experts compare the complexity of medicine to the complexity they're used to — international markets, legal issues, regulations, etc., all complicated issues for sure, but with a lot more consistency and expected outcomes. Addressing disease is very different than addressing production line complexities.

All of which is why Rescue The Doctor isn't a business training book, and isn't pretending to be. Even if we did know how to increase efficiency in medicine, the problem isn't really efficiency. The problem is on the human

---

[17] http://www.kingsfund.org.uk/blog/2012/06/can-lean-redesign-stick-health-care

side of things. It's about personal effectiveness and effectiveness with others, about leadership and not just time management. Doctors need a set of personal and people skills, and a business understanding that isn't being taught in medical school — and historically hasn't been seen as valuable for doctors. And even before doctors understand the skills they need, they have to understand that they need any new skills at all.

* * *

Doctors want to practice medicine the way they've always practiced medicine. The patient hasn't changed, thinks the doctor, so why should he? Of course, doctors have always had to change — because medicine changes. Doctors can accept when care standards change, when research changes, or when best treatments change. Internal change within medicine — doctors and researchers uncovering information that changes how to best treat patients — is something they're used to dealing with. But external change — outsiders coming in and telling doctors what to do, not always motivated by data and science — is different.

Doctors need to accept that business matters. That money is a factor in a way it never before was, and that choices are made with or without them. And that it's better for those choices to be made with doctors at the table, instead of with them outside the room, banging on the doors and windows in protest. That's all. That simple realization should be the industry's entire goal at this point, not bringing in specific systems and tools that aren't going to work because, first, medicine really is different, and, second, Old World healers who think that medicine and business must remain separate worlds are never going to let the tools work — they're never even going to give them a chance.

* * *

The truth is that management desperately wants doctors to engage. They just don't know how to get them on their side of the table. We close this section with a quote from a UK paper discussing the National Health Service, effectively summing up everything both sides ought to understand about medicine and business, and the need to come together and partner for the best solutions:

> *"Managers don't want to become more clinical, but because doctors haven't engaged, they've been forced to make more and more policy decisions, further alienating doctors. We want to bring doctors back into the model so we can stop this downward spiral. Partnership working is the way forward to ensure the strengths of both groups are deployed effectively to implement change and achieve excellence."*[18]

---

[18] http://www.healthknowledge.org.uk/public-health-textbook/organisation-management/5a-understanding-itd/interactions

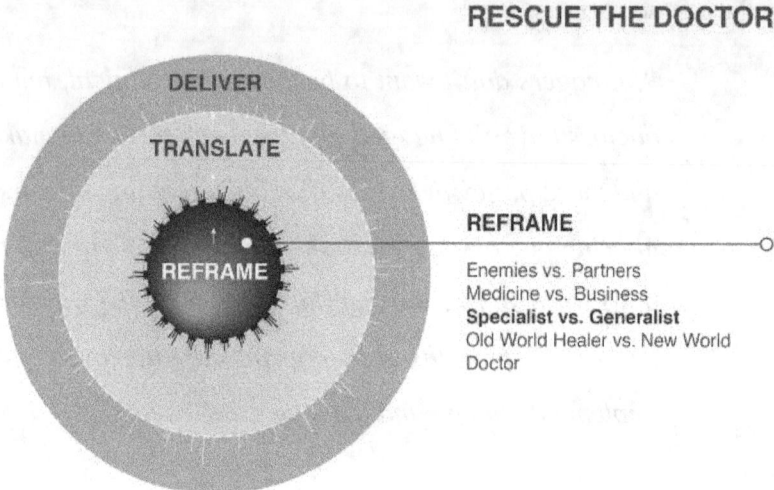

RESCUE THE DOCTOR

DELIVER
TRANSLATE
REFRAME

REFRAME

Enemies vs. Partners
Medicine vs. Business
Specialist vs. Generalist
Old World Healer vs. New World Doctor

SPECIALIST VS. GENERALIST

Doctors are used to thinking like specialists. They spend years in medical school, residency, and fellowships (often with research on top of all of that) in order to specialize and further sub-specialize in what ends up being a very, very narrow strip of health care — one organ, one disease, one condition — and the ones who don't specialize end up referring many of their patients to these specialists when the time comes. No doctor would dream of trying to treat every condition, not in a medical world as complex and detailed as we have today. An internist, for instance, would never presume to tell a surgeon what technique to use for his surgery. An internist probably wouldn't even be familiar with the options, and almost certainly wouldn't feel comfortable inserting himself into a conversation about the strengths and weaknesses of the different possible surgical approaches.

See, doctors are used to the barriers of entry for specialist conversations being very high. There is simply too much knowledge needed before you can even think you might know the answer. The dangers are too great — of hurting the patient, of being wrong, of seeming uninformed, irresponsible, incompetent. Doctors can't speculate. They either know what they're talking about, or they don't give an answer. Or at least they shouldn't give an answer.

And we're not arguing they should. On the medical side, doctors absolutely need to be specialists. The problem is when they maintain that mindset even when the conversation turns to the business side of health care. They don't engage, because they know they're not the experts. They defer, and then complain about the results. They presume that in order to be involved in the decision-making process, they need to know the same level of detail they would be expected to know when deciding about a patient's cancer treatment, or a medication dosage, and they're not interested in becoming experts in business, so they check out.

What they're missing is that in the world of business, they don't need to be specialists in order to have value. They need to wear the glasses of a generalist — and those are glasses doctors aren't used to wearing. In business, the barriers are much lower. It's not that business is simple — although compared to medicine, one could certainly make that argument. It's merely that business is not a science to the same degree that medicine is. Answers are not necessarily right or wrong. They're guesses. You can speculate, you can discuss, you can have an opinion — even if you haven't read every book there is to read and taken every class.

To have an idea about how a hospital could market itself to a new population of patients doesn't require a marketing degree. And the marketing experts certainly may know much less about how to effectively attract patients than a doctor would. The reverse is not true. Any doctor would be appalled to have a marketing expert weigh in on a treatment plan. They act as if the marketing department would feel the same way about a doctor weighing in on a new promotional campaign, but the truth is that the marketing department would likely love the doctor's input. In the Old World, doctors didn't have to get involved in these kinds of discussions — indeed, these kinds of discussions would never even happen, because what kind of hospital needed to market itself? But in the New World, a successful doctor has to be involved, as much as he can be, or risk being marginalized and ignored.

* * *

There are a small number of doctors who have business degrees. We wrote an opinion piece about business education for doctors in the *Financial Times* in late 2013. We argued that reserving discussions about business for those select few doctors who devoted years to pursuing a business degree is a terrible waste of the value that the rest of the doctor population can bring to the table. These aren't issues for the elite few to discuss. These are issues that end up mattering to all doctors, and part of rescuing themselves and the whole profession is for doctors to engage. The truth is that it's not just management that needs to learn from doctors with regard to these critical business issues — there is also a fair bit that doctors can learn by taking part in this generalist thinking.

The BMJ (formerly the British Medical Journal) published a piece in 2003 titled, "What doctors and managers can learn from each other." The points made are even more relevant today, as another decade has passed of doctors and managers acting like enemies instead of partners.

> *"Doctors are, I believe, losing out in modern healthcare systems because of their discomfort with leadership, strategy, systems thinking, negotiation, genuine team working,*

organisational development, economics, and finance. Learning more about these things from managers, their colleagues, may make them not only more effective but happier, less lost within modern health care." [19]

This is the crux of the specialist-generalist problem. Too often, doctors are remaining purposefully ignorant about business. They fear that in order to understand these issues, they have to be an accountant or go to business school. That isn't true. Peter made this mistake, spending years trying to be an expert *instead of simply diving in*. Doctors don't need to be the experts on these issues. They merely need to know enough to participate, and be able to *work with the experts*.

When doctors complain to us that management has taken over and is now dictating what they can and cannot do, what it says to us is that the doctors have forgotten why management came along in the first place. Management, finance, accounting — they are all meant to be support staff. They are there to serve the doctors, to help institutions achieve their goals, and put doctors' plans into action. It is when they are asked to do more than support — when they are forced to take the lead and make all of the decisions, because the doctors refuse to engage — that the problems typically begin. Management can't support a medical team that won't talk to them, that wants to defer all responsibility to them and then complain when they don't agree with the decisions. Doctors can't have it both ways — they can't abdicate responsibility and then throw a fit when things don't turn out the way they want.

Peter spent ten years reading business books, attending lectures, workshops, and conferences. The same level of engagement and detail he would pay to a new neurological disease he wanted to become an expert in.

---

[19] http://www.ncbi.nlm.nih.gov/pmc/articles/PMC1125519/

But generalists don't need to do that. They don't need to look at the forest with a magnifying glass. They just need to look up and see the trees.

* * *

We're not saying doctors should stop thinking like specialists. They still need to be specialists in medicine. They just need to make sure they're using the right mindset when they're thinking about other issues. It's hard when you've spent your entire training learning how to think like a specialist. It's hard when generalist thinking is neither encouraged nor practiced. It's hard to switch back and forth, and figure out how much you really need to know about business in order to engage. That's why we wrote this book. Doctors don't have these skills, and that's a big part of why the profession is suffering.

Fewer than 4% of hospitals in the United States are headed by doctors, as compared to 35% in 1935. That's from an article in Academic Medicine, titled "Educating Physicians to Lead Hospitals." Not all doctors want to lead hospitals — most go into medicine to be clinicians, not to sit in an office and never see patients — but the ones who do have those skills and those interests are not getting a chance to grow into those roles.

> *"Some may argue that hospital leadership is simply not part of a physician's job description. 'I went to medical school to learn to care for the sick,' a physician may say, 'not to read financial statements, study organization charts, lobby community leaders, and develop strategic plans.' ... Yet physicians pay a high price for remaining on the sidelines of*

> *hospital leadership. Career satisfaction in the medical profession is deteriorating."*[20]

Indeed, it is critical to note, according to the Institute for the Study of Labor, "hospitals positioned higher in the US News and World Report's Best Hospitals ranking are led disproportionately by physicians."[21] This is why it is so crucial for doctors to start thinking like generalists — for the good of themselves, and for the good of their institutions. Having more doctors able to engage, and potentially open to leadership positions, will make things better for the entire profession, and be a critical way to cope with the change from Old World to New World medicine.

---

[20] http://journals.lww.com/academicmedicine/fulltext/2009/10000/perspective__educating_physicians_to_lead.16.aspx

[21] http://ftp.iza.org/dp5830.pdf

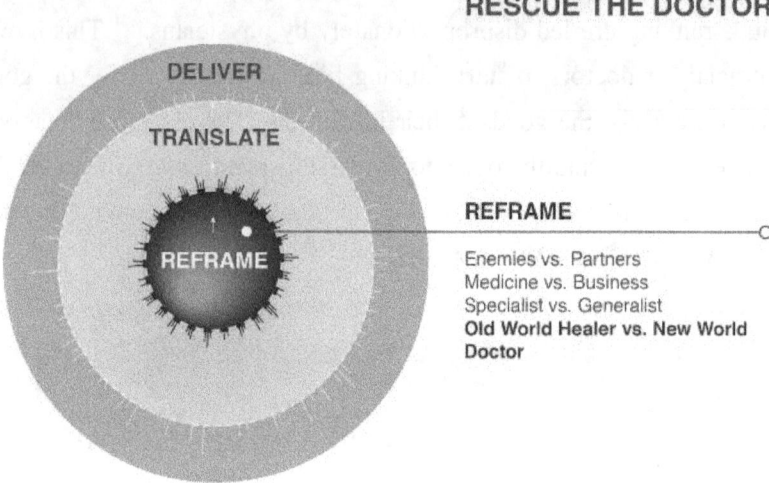

OLD WORLD HEALER VS. NEW WORLD DOCTOR

It used to be that being a good doctor meant being a good clinician. It was all about the medicine. But no longer is merely being a good clinician enough. The U.K.'s General Medical Council writes:

> *"Being a good doctor means more than simply being a good clinician. Every day, doctors provide leadership to their colleagues, and vision for the organisations in which they work and to the profession as a whole."*[22]

---

[22] http://www.gmc-uk.org/guidance/ethical_guidance/management_for_doctors.asp

The popular culture puts on a pedestal doctors who can pluck an obscure diagnosis from thin air. Dr. Gregory House — the title character of the American medical drama, *House* — is a terrible colleague, miserable to work with, headstrong and stubborn. But he has a knack for stumbling on the right diagnosis, and so he is the hero. It works on television, but not in the New World of medicine. In the Old World, Dr. House might be called "the best," but in the New World, we need to radically rethink the definition of what "best" means.

Frankly, "the best" is a pretty meaningless idea in the New World. As we've said, no doctor can possibly be "the best" at everything. Medicine is far too complicated for that. "The best" doctor for most patients is a team of doctors — and not just doctors, but nurses and an administrative team on their side as well. You can have "the best" surgeon, but if no one's making sure the operating room is on schedule, and no one's ordered the right instruments, and the power goes out during the surgery, being "the best" doesn't mean much.

What you want in the New World is a team that communicates, that trusts each other, and that can work together effectively and safely. Yes, you want doctors who are experts in medicine — but that's a given, and it's not enough. In the Old World, we had a star system. The best doctor was a star. We still promote that way of thinking — in the U.S., magazines list the annual "best doctors," but it's a meaningless title bestowed to doctors who pay to be listed or who encourage their patients to vote for them, as if practicing medicine is like being a contestant on a reality show. Those doctors — competing to land on those lists, to be called "the best" — are often the ones feeling most disaffected as health care changes, because those accolades they've been chasing their entire careers no longer really matter. Charisma and image aren't nearly enough — it's about character and collaboration. Management doesn't want *lone healers*. They want good colleagues, with the skill to navigate the system and work well with others.

* * *

We hear your skepticism. *You can go on and on about how the hospital wants team players, but I don't care that much about my hospital — I care about my patients. And my patients need a doctor with the answers, not just a doctor who the managers and nurses all want to have lunch with.*

That may have been true in the Old World. But the fact is that *you don't get to keep treating your patients if you don't have those other skills too.* They're going to take your patients away. They're going to put someone else in your office who plays well with others and doesn't make it harder to run the hospital than it already is. You can't hide in your office and insist that what makes a good doctor hasn't changed, and you're going to keep doing things the way you've always done them. That's what has gotten you into this mess, and created this hole you're desperate to dig your way out of. The answer isn't doing things the way you've always done them. The answer is understanding what is changing, and getting ahead of the curve. What it means to be a good doctor in the New World is different, very different, than what it meant before. You don't have the luxury of ignoring it.

It's not just that the hospital doesn't want stars anymore. Being a star these days is virtually impossible.

We've talked about specialization. What does it even mean to be a star when your specialty is so narrow that no one outside of it has heard of you? Your colleagues don't know or care who the best at your sub-sub-specialty is. They wouldn't even know how to ascertain the answer. What they care about — what they notice — is whether you show up at meetings, keep your promises, and give doctors a bad name in the eyes of the support staff you all have to work with. They're looking for a broader contribution.

Technology has also made the star system part of an antiquated past. The machines can see things at a molecular level, in far more detail than a doctor ever could on his own. Your differentiator can't just be your diagnostic skills when technology can do it even better than you can.

Standardized treatment plans, checklists, evidence-based medicine all mean that being a star clinician means less and less. Everyone is following the same protocol. What distinguishes you in the New World are your relationships, your people skills, your integrity, your credibility and character, and your ability to work as a member of a top-notch team — not merely your knowledge of the latest research.

And who gets the promotion? The team player, not the individual achiever. The movement from the Old World to the New World is a movement from Old World *lone healers* to New World doctors who focus on the entire health care system. From your focus being on one patient to your focus being on your entire institution and how you can make things better for every patient who walks through the door. It's absolutely frustrating for doctors who've grown up in a system where knowing the answer as soon as you're called on has been the ultimate test of competence since medical school — but in some ways, it can incredibly freeing. The path to success isn't just knowing more, faster. There are other ways to be valuable, and other ways to advance. You don't have to be the surgeon with the best hands. You can be the surgeon with the second-best hands, who everyone wants to work with — and you move up the ranks just as quickly, if not even more so.

* * *

The model isn't the same as it used to be. According to McKinsey, "[health care] needs fewer component providers who specialize in a single task, such as taking diagnostic images. Instead, it will need more healers (providers who can achieve specific objectives for patients during episodes of care) and partners (providers who can help improve a patient's health and wellness over a longer period of time)."[23] That's a different set of skills, and

---

[23] http://www.mckinsey.com/Insights/Health_systems_and_services/ Claiming_the_1_trillion_prize_in_US_health_care?cid=other-eml-alt-mip-mck-oth-1309

a set of skills it takes new training to be comfortable with. None of it means you don't also have to be great at medicine. Of course you're not a good doctor if you're not great at medicine. It just means there is more to it than that.

A smart institution isn't going to want a collection of the best at medicine. It's going to fill its ranks the way a general manager of a sports franchise will fill his team's roster. Just like a team needs a player at every position, a hospital needs people in every role — leaders, strategic thinkers, people who can execute, mentors, communicators, and more. Not everyone needs to do everything, but people need to fill those roles in addition to their jobs as clinicians. You need to be what we like to call a doctor-plus — someone who brings some skills to the table beyond the medicine, and helps the institution be something greater than the sum of its parts. All of those plusses that you and your colleagues bring beyond the clinical expertise is what makes your institution able to survive and thrive in the new health care world. It's as simple as that.

Unfortunately, the way doctors are trained and recruited does not yet reflect this new reality. The problem with medical education, as we see it, is that, in almost all cases, the admissions process is not searching for doctors with these other skills, and the education certainly isn't teaching them. We're in a New World of medicine but doctors are still being trained and prepared for the Old World. That's why there is so much dissatisfaction and burnout. "The doctors' power rests on their professional prestige," writes *The Economist*, "rather than managerial acumen, for which they are neither selected nor trained."[24]

In our *Financial Times* article, we wrote that across the world, the medical school curriculum is focused almost exclusively on diagnosis and treatment. Doctors learn how to heal, but not how to practice. The nuts and bolts of working as a doctor — dealing with staff, setting up an office,

---

[24] http://www.economist.com/node/21556227

managing a budget with ever-increasing demands, the commercial realities of the real world — are not just ignored but we believe are deliberately removed from a doctor's training, seen as tarnishing the purity of patient care.

In a perfect world, this is not a bad thing. We want doctors to be focused on patient care above all else. But the institutions where doctors are practicing are forced to think about profit even when the doctors themselves do not. If the doctors don't worry about these issues, someone else has to. And that someone else is going to take power and autonomy away from doctors.

If we start to train New World doctors, who understand these issues, we can end up with hospitals that are run not by management, but in fact by doctors — *teams* of doctors who all bring unique and complementary skills to the table. And this will improve medicine and prevent doctors from burnout.

These doctor-plus skills have long been ignored — they've been undervalued, under-recognized, and underappreciated. Doctors haven't been rewarded for their business skills, their relationship skills, the soft human skills — when dealing with people beyond their patients — that are so vitally important in this New World of medicine. These are the skills doctors need in order to be happy, successful, and satisfied in the New World. These are the skills that we focus on as we help you *translate* and *deliver*, giving you what you need to go from an Old World healer to a New World doctor, regain control over your career, and rise in the ranks.

This is what we've been trying to say in the entire *reframe* section: *a great percentage of the problems that doctors are facing have nothing to do with the traditional measures of clinical competency.* The pain points revolve around the human aspect, dealing with others in their daily interactions. What makes a good doctor, now, more than ever, is having the skills — on top of the clinical pre-requisites — to cope with these New World challenges. *Doctors* need to be the leaders. *Doctors* need to be the connectors between management and patients, between research and clinics — the translational bridge that carries medicine from the Old World into the New.

In the next section of the book, we move from reframing how you see the world to helping you translate this vision into your everyday reality. There is a core set of skills that you can learn — quickly and easily — that can change the way you approach your professional life and lead you and your institution toward rescue. These four drivers — Enemies vs. Partners, Medicine vs. Business, Specialist vs. Generalist, and Old World Healer vs. New World Doctor — are changing and have already changed the profession, but it is not a lost cause for doctors still seeing the world the way they've always seen it. You can be rescued, and the entire profession can be rescued. It is within each doctor's power, and within each doctor's control.

TRANSLATE

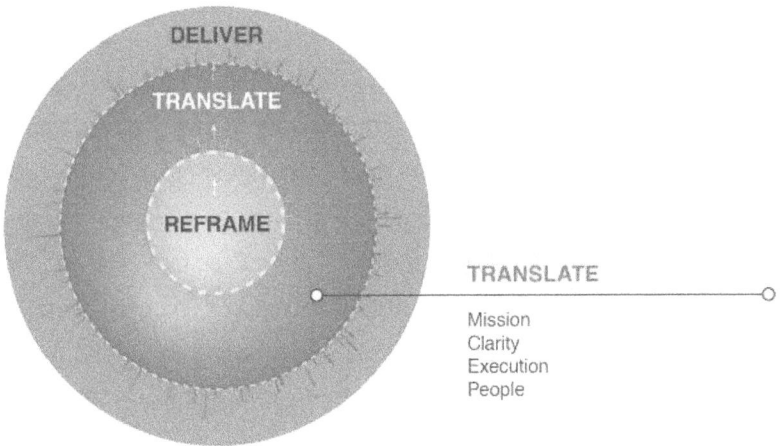

Think about the doctors you know — the ones you trained with, the ones you work with, the ones you only see from afar, at meetings or conferences, and the ones you only hear about, from patients or from colleagues. Think about the ones you read about, the ones who seem to have it all, who don't appear to be struggling the same way the rest of the profession is. Think about the doctors whose careers you can sometimes find yourself envious of, the ones who are universally known, respected, and even loved — by their patients, by their teams, and by their institutions. The ones who seem like pillars of the profession, examples of what a doctor is and can still be in our society.

How have some doctors seemed to escape the problems we talked about in the first part of this book? How have some doctors thrived even as their colleagues struggle? How have some doctors in fact used the changes in the profession to their advantage, and built their careers to great heights even as health care has been fighting through transformation and even turmoil?

Of course part of the answer is that what you see from the outside isn't always the reality of what someone's life is truly like. The very same doctors who seem like they have it all may well be struggling to cope with the drivers we've already described — they may simply be hiding it better than most.

But the ones who truly have transcended these issues and are making the most of the uncertainty and change? You probably realize it isn't just about their clinical skills. Sure, it's possible that some of the best at transitioning to the New World are also top clinicians, and are standing out because of their excellence in medicine. More likely, it's an entirely different set of skills that has powered their rise. It's not a set of skills doctors are taught in medical school, but it's also not a set of skills that can't be taught. And while it seems like knowing how to cope with change, take control of your destiny, work effectively with others, and reach the levels of satisfaction and acclaim that you strive for are skills that you either have or don't — or that it's all based on luck that can't be forced or manufactured — to think this way is simply wrong.

You *can* be the kind of doctor that others think about when they ask themselves who the leaders are in the profession, who has it all figured out, who is making the most of this time of great transformation and change. You *can* be a New World Doctor. What it takes is not rocket science, and it's not better medicine. We trust that your clinical skills are strong. What it takes is translating the issues in the first section of the book into concrete practices to bring you from the Old World to the New World. What it takes is a set of skills that isn't taught but can be learned. What it takes is first committing to the **mission** of being a rescued doctor, and then applying three bits of knowledge we will talk about in this section of the book — gaining **clarity**, fine-tuning your **execution**, and optimizing your work with the **people** around you, building effective relationships and bringing them with you on your journey to the New World.

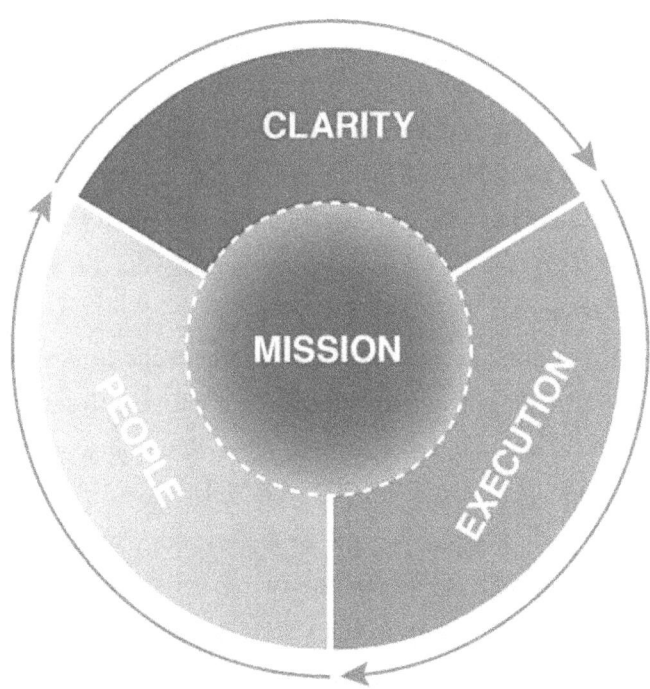

In this section of the book, we will translate the big changes in health care into these skills that you as doctors need in order to become leaders in the New World. We will show you how to move from looking through Old World eyes into seeing a New World view. Too many doctors don't have enough awareness of these critical skills. It's not your fault — you were taught what you needed to know when being a doctor was just about knowing medicine. But medicine is no longer enough.

That's right. Medicine is no longer enough.

To an Old World healer, this surely sounds like blasphemy. Medicine has been for so much of history the beginning and the end of what it means to be a doctor. What more could there possibly be for a doctor to know than medicine? The two words, 'doctor' and 'medicine,' are so intertwined with each other in our minds that it seems like a question that no one would even think to ask. If you know medicine, you are a doctor. If you are a doctor, you know medicine. And in the Old World, the conversation ended there. But if the first section of this book illustrated anything, it should be that medicine is more complex than it used to be and there are new questions we have to ask if we want to survive, thrive, and lead as doctors — if we want to be rescued.

The Old World mission of a doctor-healer was easy to explain. You become a doctor to help and heal patients. That is all you spend your time and energy on, and if you do it well, you are a successful doctor. There is no other measuring stick in the Old World.

The New World mission is of course also to help and heal patients — doctors don't become doctors without that drive to contribute to society. But, now, understanding the changing world we've been describing, you have to embrace the idea that in the New World, your mission as a doctor goes beyond just helping your patients. To get from the Old World to the New World, you need to embrace a broader mission — as a system healer, not just a one-on-one patient healer, and as a doctor who must constantly grow his own capabilities and skills as a leader of the profession, and not just someone who can devote one hundred percent of his time to office visits, practicing the same kind of medicine he has practiced for decades.

This section of the book is about making the commitment to invest in yourself, to invest in your institution, and to invest in the people around you. It's about saying "yes" to change, "yes" to growth, and "yes" to the New World.

* * *

Look, doctors are getting burned out because they're saying "no." They're saying "no" to change. They're saying "no" to growth. They're saying "no" to the business and finance professionals leading their institutions, saying "no" to the new expectations of a doctor, saying "no" to the New World. They're trying to hide, or they're trying to run, and those are not winning strategies. The world is changing with or without you. You can only rescue yourself — and rescue health care — by saying "yes."

With a strong and powerful "yes," you enter this section of the book ready to translate your work as a doctor from the Old World to the New World, ready to embrace a new set of ideas about **clarity** over your goals and the goals of your institution, about the day-to-day **execution** of your responsibilities as a New World doctor, and about working with the **people** around you, growing relationships and growing leaders. This is your mission in the New World: to invest in yourself, your institution, and your colleagues — and, in doing so, rescue yourself and rescue health care.

The rest of this *translate* section will give you the knowledge you need to be a rescued doctor. Then, in the *deliver* section, we'll put everything together and show you how to actually achieve results — to put Rescue The Doctor into practice and effect real change. But before you can effect change, you need to embrace the three skills that follow. Only then can you truly transform your professional life — and your institution.

RESCUE THE DOCTOR

CLARITY

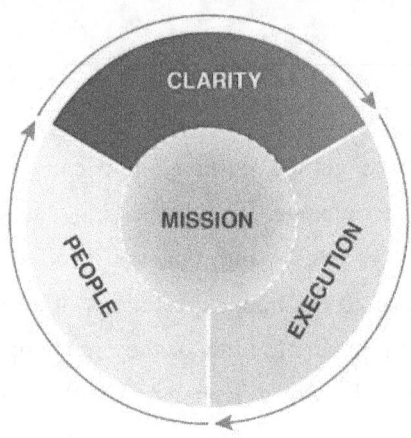

CLARITY: "SET THE COURSE"

What will your organization look like in five years? Where will you fit in that organization, and what will your role be? Who will determine your professional future, and what the care of your patients will look like — and what are their goals?

These aren't the kinds of questions doctors typically ask themselves, or the kinds of questions they seek answers to from the people around them. After all, patients keep coming, whether or not you ask these questions, and whether or not you spend any time worrying about where you fit in the broader world of health care. You're a doctor — of course there will always will be a place for you. But that's not where the thinking should end.

In our busy, ultra-scheduled day-to-day professional lives, few of us ever spend much time considering the bigger picture. We have our battles at work over details — and they're often details that are critically important, and we're not trying to minimize those concerns — but, as we considered when looking at *Enemies vs. Partners* in the previous section of the book, we don't often take the time to truly understand where someone else is coming from, what's motivating him, and what's driving the decisions he's making.

It's both a blessing and a curse that doctors, for the most part, haven't needed to tackle the kinds of things that people in most industries wrestle with every day, about goals and direction, roles and responsibilities, needs and purposes. Patients do keep coming, whether or not you're thinking about your goals or the goals of your institution. Your hospital will continue to exist (you hope), and you will continue to be employed. You'll be judged against certain benchmarks (or, sometimes, none at all), and as long as you don't do something spectacularly unfortunate, your professional world will continue to spin — and you will continue to be busy, tired, and intellectually and emotionally drained by the end of each day.

But, as you're already seeing, or you wouldn't have picked up this book, without thinking about these larger issues, your career will drift away from you, and health care will continue drifting away from doctors and into the hands of the people who do spend their time considering these kinds of things, looking at the bigger picture, understanding the needs of all of health care's new stakeholders, and working to meet them.

Some doctors avoid the larger questions because you don't see yourselves as empowered to effect change in your institution. And it's true that in the Old World, doctors didn't have to get involved in the larger issues facing hospitals and facing the profession as a whole. Clarity was a fairly easy concept. You merely needed to think about what your patients wanted, keep up with the latest research (which was only published in a handful of places), and as new procedures and tools came onto the market, quickly pick up whatever knowledge you needed. Your area of concern didn't need to stretch beyond, to the bigger discussions swirling around health care — in fact, there were few if any bigger discussions swirling around health care, back when health care wasn't so complex.

But the world now is very different. You're at the center of one of the largest industries out there, a huge part of virtually every country's economy, with the cost increasing every day. Health care is at the top of the agenda for so many diverse groups — those who consume it, provide it, pay for it, and profit from it. The amount of money being spent is so vast that countries can't afford to get it wrong, with aging populations needing more and more care, and the cost of equipment, procedures, medication, and research escalating every day. Doctors are the ones with the knowledge to help — with the medical expertise to know how to sort through the options and allocate money and resources most effectively for patients — and it's critical that you are part of the discussion.

The problem is that you can't be a useful part of the discussion without knowing how the industry works, what the people around you care about, and what your institution is trying to accomplish. Clarity is about taking the steps to gain the knowledge that can make you a contributor to the discussion, an ally for your institution, and an informed doctor acting not only in the best interests of your patients but in the best interests of your institution and the health care system as a whole — which, ultimately, will lead to better long-term outcomes for your patients because you will still have a functioning, successful hospital in which to practice, and the resources to provide them with the best possible care.

* * *

In practice, Clarity means asking the right questions of the right people, with the goal of understanding the landscape around you. Where does the budget of your institution come from? Who are the key decision-makers within your organization, and what are their goals? Who are the key influencers outside your organization, and what are their needs? What is the agenda of the hospital managers, of the finance department, of the politicians with their eyes on your institution, and of any other stakeholders who care about the work you do? What do your patients want, and are you effectively providing it? What is your hospital aiming to supply to the community, and are they succeeding at doing so?

The answers to these questions aren't always easy, and often require real conversations between you and people in your organization you may not always reach out to, or see eye-to-eye with. But they are conversations that a doctor needs to have in order to rescue himself, because these conversations are the only way to start building the bridge back from Doctor Island and restore your place as a leader with control over your professional destiny. It's only after you understand the needs of the people around you that you can more fully see how you fit into the present and future of your organization, and where you can best be of service.

* * *

This is obviously very different from what a doctor needed to concern himself with in the Old World. It requires a fundamental change in thinking about your role and about your responsibility to your institution. It requires fully embracing your new mission as a system-focused professional, and fully committing to the idea of being a New World doctor. All three of the skills we're discussing in this section require real change in terms of how you think about your job, and for each skill we want to look at the traditional views and how they must be translated to the New World. We will then explore each skill a bit more deeply, in trying to figure out how you can best apply it to your life.

CLARITY

OLD WORLD VIEWS	NEW WORLD VIEWS
I don't need to think about the pressures facing my organization or its key stakeholders — my stakeholders are my patients.	I have so many stakeholders, each with their own agenda — and it is critical to my work that I understand who they are and what they want.
My future is the same as my present — I treat patients.	My future involves being a patient healer, but also a system healer, helping patients (and the community) navigate the increasing complexity.
The important learning I must do as a doctor is stay up to date on treatments and research.	The important learning I must do includes a familiarity with the entire health care world so I can know how to best help my patients.
I am insulated from business concerns, because there will always be sick patients and there will always be jobs for doctors.	Hospitals close, budgets get cut, and business realities absolutely matter in medicine, even if I'd like to believe they don't.

DISCUSSION: DOCTORS AS MEDIATORS OF THE HEALTH CARE SYSTEM

It may have caught your eye in the New World views above — the word "mediator," and doctors now forced to see their role as mediators of the health care system, the link between the system and your patients. We think this is particularly important to focus on as you make your journey from the Old World to the New World, because it's very different from how most doctors have traditionally seen themselves. The *lone healer* model is in many ways the polar opposite of the mediator model: as a *lone healer*, solutions are all about you; as a mediator, solutions are about connecting your patients to what they need, whether that means inside your office or elsewhere.

Solutions to health care problems have become so much more varied and complex than they used to be — at both the micro level and the macro level. But what they all have in common is that they are filtered through doctors. Your role in the New World is to help your patients — and, for that matter, all of your stakeholders — navigate this complex system. Which means that your job goes far beyond being a clinician. Your Old World colleagues are fighting against this idea instead of embracing it. They're hiding from it, pretending the world hasn't changed.

They're keeping themselves in the dark about the range of things their colleagues and their institutions are doing — but if you don't have complete knowledge of what is going on around you, it is impossible to serve as an effective mediator for your patients and point them in the right direction. You must understand what is happening all around you to truly help your patients — and help the patients who might be sent by others to you, from every direction. You must transfer your caring from your own individual patients to the entire patient system, and help others build new capabilities. This is your New World role.

A WHOLE NEW CONCEPT OF CUSTOMERS

You're used to thinking of your customers as exclusively your own patients. That's just not the case in the New World. Every patient is potentially your customer — but it goes beyond that. All of the key stakeholders are your customers. Management and administrators, finance, politicians — all of the so-called enemies we talked about in the *reframe* section are your customers, and it is your job to understand them and help them to understand you. The stakeholders in business and finance are looking to improve the efficiency of the entire system. If you don't understand what they are trying to do, and the issues they are thinking about, you can't possibly help them make better decisions — and then nothing will change. With your medical expertise — something they don't have — you can help them make better decisions for your patients, but it's only by finding out how they see the world and understanding the pressures they face that you can truly become someone they can rely on, someone who can see the situation from all of the different angles, and someone who can really contribute.

The truth is that Old World healers don't fully appreciate the complexity of the system and how many interests they need to serve. It is not until you actually start to interact with all of the stakeholders you've been avoiding up to this point that you will realize how complex the health care industry has become. And you'll also become more and more adept at navigating this growing complexity, coordinating care for your patients, and advocating for them in all the right ways.

THE PARTICULAR CHALLENGE OF FINANCE

When we talk about clarity regarding finances, it's so easy to throw up your hands and walk away. The knee-jerk reaction of virtually every doctor we talk to is that all finance wants to do is cut the budget, take things away from the doctor, and make our jobs more difficult. Truth is, finance needs you. They need you to achieve their ultimate goal, which is to have a financially secure, high-performing hospital. Ultimately, if your hospital isn't financially secure, it will be at risk — of losing funds, of losing resources, perhaps even closing down. That serves no one — not you, and not your patients.

The secret that finance professionals keep telling us is that far from reducing services, what finance really wants is for you to do your job as well as you can. What's getting in the way of a financially secure hospital often isn't the services the doctors are providing, but fines, court cases, penalties — expenses entirely outside the clinical world that doctors care most about. But most doctors won't engage long enough to understand this. And the finance people end up having to make choices without the doctors guiding their hands. You need to engage. You need to talk to them and find out what their priorities are, what outcomes they are looking for — and then work with them to get there. That's what clarity is all about.

CLARITY IN BUSINESS IS NOT THE SAME AS CLARITY IN MEDICINE

We talk to many doctors who worry about engaging with finance and other stakeholders outside of their medical specialty. They know the barrier to entry in medicine is high — the amount of training you need to make a contribution as a clinician is massive, of course — and they assume that same barrier to entry exists for every discipline. But it doesn't. You don't need to be an expert in business to engage in those discussions and be part of the leadership team at your institution.

Business is not evidence-based in the same way medicine is. There isn't the same body of research, and the business world changes faster than people are able to act. Having an opinion based on your experience — even if you have no evidence beyond that experience — is okay. Having an idea — without knowing if it will work — is okay. It's challenging for doctors to play in a space that permits guessing and doesn't always value expertise. It's a new language, and the expectations are very different than they are in medicine.

We don't mean to say that all doctors are completely ignorant about business. Many of you run private practices and do know how business works in that sense — but that's on a small scale where you're in charge. You're used to being in charge. And so you struggle inside a large system where you don't control the ultimate decision — but that's why it's so critical to stop and listen, learn the basics, understand what others need and what they're asking for. Align yourself with your organization. Understand its goals and strategy and do what you can to set your agenda to match. That is ultimately what clarity is: aligning your direction with your organization's and setting off on that journey together.

Of course, setting the right direction is only the beginning. You actually have to work to turn your plans into reality. The next skill — Execution — will focus on the day-to-day, and the granular steps you need to take in order to move from goals to concrete progress, and how you ought to think about the way you spend your time.

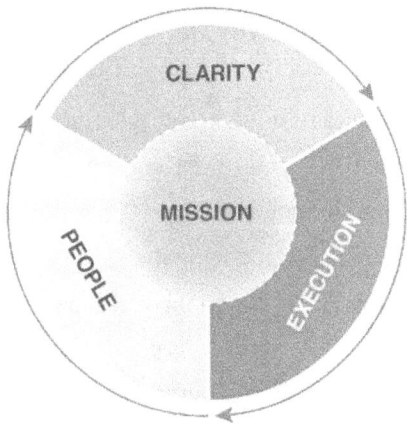

EXECUTION: "DO WHAT COUNTS"

It's one thing to know where you want to be going. It's quite another to actually do the work to get there. You can be committed to change and have a clear vision of what you need to accomplish — but if you don't actually put the right plan in place, take command of your day, and manage how you spend your time, it's very hard to ever get there. Doctors don't generally have a problem getting things done — and getting them done quickly, especially when the urgency of the situation demands it. But it's easy to confuse an ability to put out fires with the skill to balance short-term emergencies with long-term strategic planning, and end each week having accomplished something on both fronts. If

Clarity was about self-leadership, *Execution* is about self-management — focusing your attention on the right activities instead of always just the ones that are calling your name the loudest.

EXECUTION: OLD WORLD VS. NEW WORLD

If you take some time to think about what you actually spend your day doing — minute to minute — you might end up surprised. So often, we see ourselves as busy — and we genuinely are — but at the end of the day, little of substance has actually been accomplished. Sure, we spend some of our time on what's important, but we also have the paperwork, the e-mails, the meetings, the wasted time. There are always last-minute demands, emergencies that take us away from what we'd ideally like to be doing — or know we ought to be doing, but can never quite get around to working on. As doctors especially, we respond to the needs of others so much more than we get to generate our own agendas; we're so used to helping people that it's hard to say no when someone is asking. And while it's the nature of the job, it's also something we need to be aware of, and sometimes fight against in order to be true leaders and engineer change. We, more than people in most other professions, are at particular risk of spending so much of our time bouncing from one person's demands to the next — urgent and also less-urgent demands, from patients, colleagues, and others — that we may never get to those items lingering on our to-do lists that we know we need to take care of, but never quite rise to the level of urgency that ensures they get done.

Not to mention — even on those rare occasions when we do have some time to finally attack our own agenda, we're likely drained after a long day filled with the kinds of stress that comes with the work we spend most of our day doing. Whether it's dealing with urgent medical needs of our patients or just the normal stream of requests and demands, clinical work takes a lot of mental energy and focus. We don't necessarily have the stamina to then go and tackle the long-range plans, the strategic imperatives, improving "the system" for future patients and future doctors — the kind of work we all dream of being able to do, but never get around to. Skipping one day is of course not a problem — but the days add up, and before we know it, the things we realize are most important when we plan end up being the things that we never accomplish when we act.

In the Old World, this was not necessarily a problem — in the Old World, we didn't necessarily have to plan beyond the emergencies of the day. But in the New World, looking beyond your own practice and your own patients is critical. And when those vital New World concerns get ignored, you end up marooned on Doctor Island, losing control over your future, and pushed to the sidelines of medicine. You end up disaffected and burned out and everything we are trying to help you avoid with this book. You cannot succeed without a laser-sharp focus on your execution, without a commitment to getting the right things done — this week, this month, this year — because to let yourself wait until tomorrow often means letting yourself wait until a thousand tomorrows have passed and ultimately waiting forever.

EXECUTION

OLD WORLD VIEWS	NEW WORLD VIEWS
A doctor's chief obligation is to respond to medical emergencies — everything else has to come later.	I need to make time for strategic activities beyond just emergencies — particularly because those activities may be able to prevent emergencies in the future.
If I am busy being a good clinician, I have neither the time nor energy to waste on "thinking," "planning," or "reflecting."	I must make the time to think and plan and reflect because ultimately what emerges from time spent on these activities will help my patients — and help me remain effective and fulfilled as a doctor.
Patients come first, and patients always need me — to divert my attention elsewhere robs my patients of my services.	My job is not just to help my patients today, but to build a system that can help even more patients in the future.

DISCUSSION: NOT ENOUGH TIME

The number one complaint we hear from doctors we talk to is that there simply isn't enough time in the day to get everything done. Worrying about long-term goals is wonderful in the abstract, but when you're facing a waiting room full of patients, a call list a mile long, colleagues who need to talk to you, piles of paperwork, meetings, deadlines, pharmaceutical reps knocking on your door, patient families cornering you in the halls, residents, nurses, patients, all asking questions, beepers going off, e-mails to answer, and so much more (phew!) — only a superhero can possibly still have time to think about a strategic vision for the future, or all of those goals one might have set out to accomplish when worrying about *Clarity*. You'd love to see your patients and also serve on committees, tackle new projects, build your hospital a new wing with your own two hands — but there are only so many hours in the day, and, quite frankly, you may also have things you'd like to do outside of work (including sleep a couple of hours a night).

No one would accuse a doctor of being lazy if you complain that your day is already too full without new responsibilities. Doctors are undeniably busy — and undeniably busy with things that can't be rescheduled in the same way as they can be in other professions. Being a doctor is different! In traditional business training — in classes we've attended and even taught — many of the solutions to having not enough time are fairly straightforward. And pretty useless for doctors. Turn off the beeper. Don't respond to e-mails right away. Force people who want to meet with you to make an appointment. Work from home. Good luck trying any of that in a hospital or a medical office — as if any of it was possible. The reality is that what works in a law firm isn't going to work for a doctor. Of course there are emergencies. Patients don't plan their illnesses weeks in advance. Not everything can be effectively scheduled.

But if you spend as much time as we do looking at what a doctor actually does all day, it becomes clearer that the problem isn't always that there isn't enough time. It's that some of that time really is spent doing the wrong things, and if just a little bit of attention is paid to managing the schedule, big changes can become reality. Room can indeed be made for the more strategic pieces, space can be made for investing in yourself and in others, and you can take concrete steps toward becoming a New World doctor and broadening the scope of what you accomplish. The way to get there is in part through a classical business tool known as the Time Matrix — and it's the only concrete tool we're taking the time to walk you through in this book because we think it's the most critical for rescuing yourself and others. It's also one of the few tools useful in the broader world that absolutely still applies to doctors and to medicine, and that you can truly benefit from learning about.

THE TIME MATRIX

The classic model designed to help people understand and begin to take control of their daily activities involves a four-box matrix, with urgency on one axis and importance on the other — and it divides all of our activities into four quadrants:

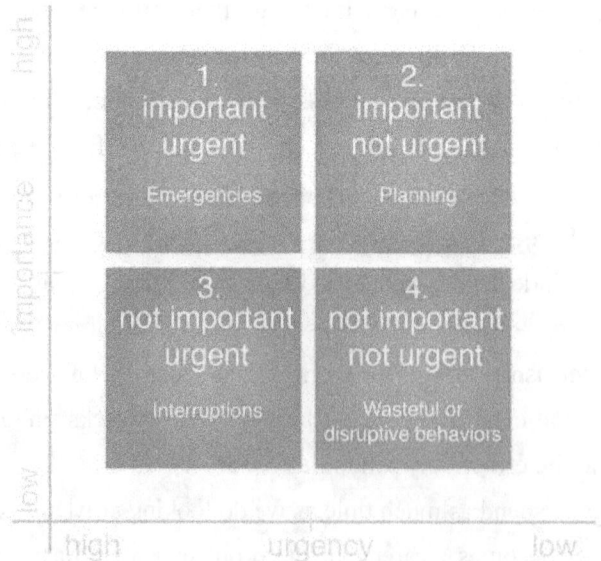

We're going to explore the matrix in some detail, but the biggest thing to remember is this: Quadrant Two is where you want to be, as much as possible. Quadrant Two is where the meaningful things happen — where you're able to take the time to think instead of just quickly reacting, where you're able to weigh options, consider long-term strategy, address problems before they grow unstoppable, and build systems to look after many patients instead of just the one standing in your office demanding your attention. Quadrant Two is about planning and strategizing, researching and reflecting, considering the future and not just the present.

In the Old World, doctors had the luxury of spending time with patients while engaged in a Quadrant Two state of mind. You could take the time to listen, to think, to plan. In the New World, there are fewer and fewer of those opportunities. With pressure to see more and more patients — and with more and more happening in your day aside from scheduled patient appointments — the kind of rewarding and productive patient interactions that doctors used to have are being replaced by a rush from one door to the next, racing through in order to meet quotas, satisfy the administration, or merely get home before midnight. Quadrant Two patient care is being replaced by Quadrant One emergency management.

At the same time as New World doctors are feeling the pressure to act in a Quadrant One mode with patients, it is also the case that — as we've been discussing — success and satisfaction as a doctor is not just about patients anymore. The kinds of things you need to do in the New World — developing relationships with colleagues and stakeholders, working on projects that improve your organization, focusing on inefficiencies and system issues, actively planning your own career and future — are all Quadrant Two activities. None of them are necessarily urgent on a day-to-day basis — but that means that they never rise to the top of the to-do list, and thus must be made a priority. Otherwise they never get done — and you can't ever make those big leaps forward that can get you out of the muck of frustration and burnout. They're the things that live in the back of your mind or the bottom of your list — but they're also the things, honestly, that separate a rescued doctor from his colleagues, and the things that you ultimately have to carve out time to do.

Instead of having the ability to spend time in Quadrant Two, it's Quadrant One — and, more troubling, Quadrants Three and Four — that end up eating most doctors' days almost entirely. Quadrant One is not hard to grasp. It's legitimate, have-to-drop-everything emergencies. Patients needing your help — the core of what you do as a doctor. But there are also endless Quadrant Three distractions in everyone's day — people demanding your attention, paperwork you must complete, meetings you must attend, situations you find yourself stuck in that are very hard to escape but not necessarily the most important things you can be doing, whether they're about patients, colleagues, management, or others. Endless e-mail chains you have to read and reply to, calls you have to make that shouldn't take as long as they do, things that ultimately aren't adding real value but have to get done as part of the job.

In a typical business workshop, they spend significant time talking about Quadrant Four waste. Playing computer games, watching television, surfing the Internet. Yes, there are doctors who do these things, but for the most part doctors aren't wasting their time on nonsense — you typically don't have the luxury, even if you wanted to. And in the Old World, we probably wouldn't be talking about Quadrant Four at all, because the practice of medicine was rewarding enough that you didn't need to find ways to distract yourself or zone out. But the New World presents lots of hidden traps, unproductive activities you can justify to yourself as useful because they're related to medicine, but in reality they're just escapes and aren't adding value. We're talking about endless research on medical sites, or reading news or stacks of journal articles not because they're necessarily useful but because you don't have the energy to do anything else. We're talking about things like playing with PowerPoint presentations beyond the point of necessity, formatting documents, trying to perfect things that don't need to be perfect. Tasks that aren't necessarily bad, but they're *not good enough*.

Why are you doing these things instead of marshalling every bit of your available time into working on the strategic Quadrant Two activities that are so important? Some of it is mindless, not really thinking about what you're doing, but some of it is stress and burnout. That stress and burnout is caused by too much time in Quadrant One, too much time in Quadrant Three, and not enough time for Quadrant Two. It's a different game in medicine than most industries. You're never going to get rid of your Quadrant One emergencies, and that shouldn't be the goal. Patients do need you, and you ought to be available to them. The issue is finding ways to wipe out as much of your Quadrant Three and Quadrant Four activities as you can, controlling the Quadrant One emergencies to the best of your ability, and getting yourself back to Quadrant Two as often as possible, being fiercely diligent about the commitments you take on, the calls you respond to, and the rabbit holes it's far too easy to fall into when you least expect it.

When outside consultants come into health care and try to use this matrix, they focus on exactly the wrong things. They don't understand that, as doctors, you can't be as rigid as people in other professions, and it's not the typical kinds of waste that bog up your day. Increased record-keeping and slavish attention paid to the clock — the typical consultant solutions — aren't what doctors need, nor is blocking some Internet sites and cutting coffee breaks a sensible piece of the equation. We know accountants can schedule their lives around tax time, and lawyers and consultants can schedule around client deadlines. But to expect doctors to be able to schedule around the bread and butter of what they do — treat their patients — is misguided at best. We're introducing the matrix not because we think it is a magic answer, but because it can get you thinking about these ideas, and the way you spend your time — and get you realizing that there is this type of Quadrant Two work that you need to prioritize, especially as a New World doctor.

GETTING OFF THE HAMSTER WHEEL

The British medical journal *BMJ* published an article a decade ago titled *Hamster Health Care*.[25]

> *"Across the globe doctors are miserable because they feel like hamsters on a treadmill. They must run faster just to stand still.... The result of the wheel going faster is not only a reduction in the quality of care but also a reduction in professional satisfaction and an increase in burn out among doctors."*

What the hamster wheel is about is that race we're talking about, that eats up so much of your day — from patient to patient, from colleague to colleague, from meeting to meeting. It's about the movement of patient care from Quadrant Two to Quadrant One, where all you get to do is put out fires, run to see the next patient, fill out form after form, go everywhere and anywhere to get to everyone who needs you. The phone is ringing, the patients are waiting — it's an adrenaline rush, sure. And it all seems important while you're doing it — necessary and even required — but it's a fleeting sense of accomplishment. At the end of the day, you barely know where the time has gone. You never get to stop and breathe, you never get to think, because you're bouncing back and forth between the emergencies and the not-so-emergencies that everyone is yelling at you about. The hustle between Quadrants One, Three, and Four — getting lost and never finding your way to Quadrant Two — can be thought of as like a Bermuda Triangle.

---

[25] BMJ. 2000 December 23; 321(7276): 1541–1542.

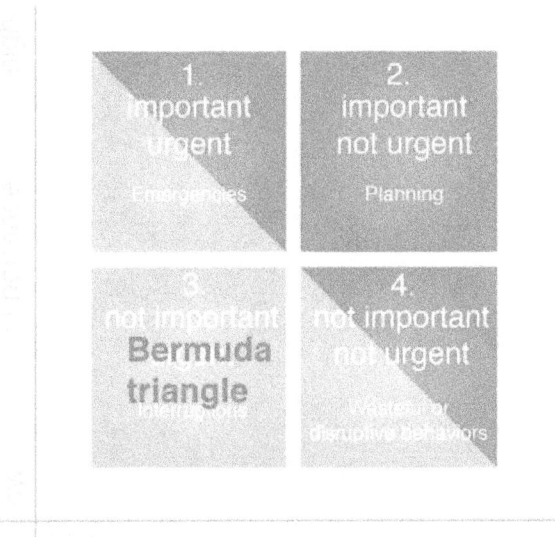

The metaphor is used in other industries — but in medicine, it's probably not the most accurate way to think about your day. You're not really caught in Quadrant Four, even if sometimes you feel like you have to escape there. What's really hurting is that bounce between Quadrants One and Three, that back-and-forth all day between the emergencies and the meetings and the paperwork and the rushed patient visits and another emergency and sixteen phone calls and thirty-four messages and yet another meeting and a stack of notes to write and one more emergency. It's everyone around you trying to grab your attention and forcing you to engage — on their schedule, not on yours. You're a ping-pong ball, caught between Quadrants One and Three, with no way to escape to what's really important for your future and the future of your organization.

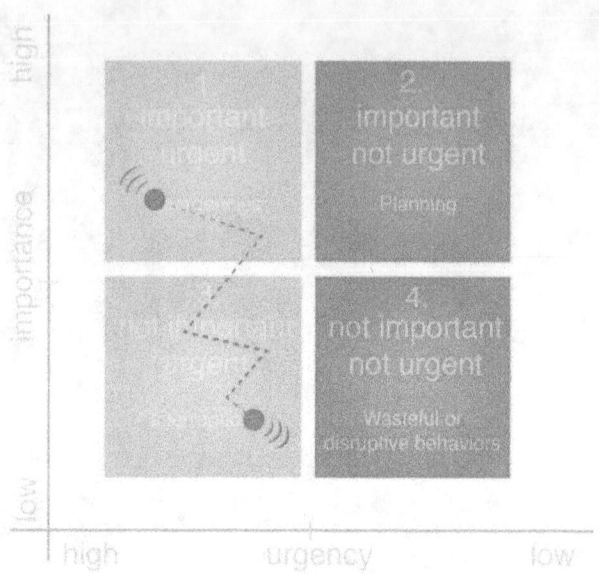

You can hope and wish all you want, but without intervention, you will never get to Quadrant Two — not because you don't want to, but because, unlike many other professions, as a doctor there just isn't a finite amount of work. *As a doctor there is always more.* Another patient will always be waiting.

How to get off the hamster wheel, and finally make it to Quadrant Two? Instead of always reacting, you have to get ahead of the game, at least when you can. You have to figure out what you can do ahead of time, what you can delegate to others, and what you might be able to eliminate entirely, in order to clear your schedule for the items that can truly make a difference. You need to take control before the phone starts ringing. Before patients start calling you, sometimes you need to call them. Get ahead of problems before they become emergencies. Think about your patients with a Quadrant Two mind, not only waiting for their Quadrant One emergencies. You can apply Quadrant Two thinking to more than you may realize. As you page through Quadrant Three paperwork, ask yourself: is there a better system for what

I'm doing? Can I help create it? There isn't always an answer, but sometimes there is, and that's the kind of thinking you need to be making an effort to engage in. As you run from one appointment to the next, ask yourself if there was a better way to meet the needs of whoever you're meeting with — and if perhaps that way wouldn't involve quite so much of your time and energy. While you address the current crisis, can you do something to improve your service for the next time this crisis occurs? Can you invest time now to save time in the future? Can you make an appointment with yourself, instead of always just making appointments with others — and find the time to do what you need to do in order to thrive?

The more effort you put into doing what matters, the more impact you will have, and the more fulfilled you will feel. But the more you spend time in Quadrant Two, the more you realize that there's a limit to what you can do alone. You can have great ideas and be doing everything you can to help yourself and your organization. But without the people around you helping and supporting you, your impact is limited. If you're able to move beyond your own silo, build strong relationships, develop the talents of others, and harness the power of those around you, the difference you make can be orders of magnitude greater.

To bring those people on that journey with you, and to expand from leadership and management of yourself to the leadership and management of others and of your entire organization, you need one final set of skills that we address in the next section, *People*. Once you add *People* to the mix, you are truly ready to deliver real change — to your own life, the lives of the people around you, and your organization as a whole.

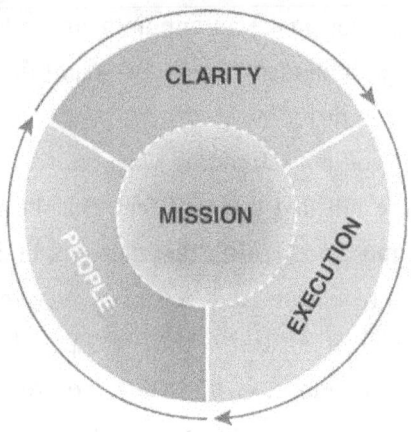

RESCUE THE DOCTOR

PEOPLE

PEOPLE: "BUILD RELATIONSHIPS — AND BUILD LEADERS"

People is about effectively and creatively collaborating with others, as well as helping others to become leaders themselves. This interpersonal leadership step moves your road to rescue from a personal victory to a true organizational victory — and gives you the skill you need to move to the last and highest level of our Rescue The Doctor program: the *delivery*.

By now you should have a clearer idea about your direction, and be thinking hard about how to truly do the things that matter most. You know what you need to accomplish. But you can't accomplish meaningful things alone. You need the help and cooperation of everyone around you — your colleagues and all of the key stakeholders in your organization. Are they partners, or are they enemies? Think about your relationships. How much genuine trust is there? Who are the people you count on and who count on you? Are you aiming for everyone to come out a winner, or do you find yourself looking at everything as a battle, with people staking out positions on both sides, fighting for someone's defeat?

As doctors, you aren't necessarily used to relying on others — the *lone healer* model is still rearing its head, after all. We'd be naïve to say it's all about honesty and better communication and leave it there — there's a history that needs to be overcome, a pattern that so many doctors have fallen into, that we've been discussing throughout this book. Doctors haven't made it easy for managers and everyone else they deal with who doesn't wear a white coat. Many can be difficult, defensive, and stubborn at times — not entirely the doctors' fault (managers have made their own difficult choices as well) but doctors do have to absorb some of the blame.

The good news is that broken relationships can almost always be fixed. You can overcome a troubled history merely by putting in some effort. Compared to what goes on in most hospitals, any effort at all is, quite frankly, a huge step, and a step that the people around you will notice, appreciate, and respect.

It's not optional in the New World to get along with others and work with them to improve the entire patient system. You need to effectively engage with the people you deal with — and you need to build champions to join you in the New World of health care. What is a champion? Someone open to change, who you can bring on your journey and who can help you make a difference. Someone you see as a potential leader and who you want to help grow into a rescued doctor just like you. You need to be the kind of person that can grow these champions, a person that others want to work with, learn from, and follow — and then you need to help those people better themselves, building the next generation of leadership and sustaining your organization for the future.

In the Old World, the focus was often limited to short-term results — who were the people who could help the organization today, help solve a specific problem or fill a specific role? Those people are still valuable in the New World, but they're not the only people you need to watch for. You also need to build the next generation of leaders so that the organization can sustain its improvement, and keep getting better. It's a different way of seeing your organization, and your responsibility toward it — you're not just dealing with what services you can provide your patients today, but you need to keep an eye on tomorrow, and making sure the right people are in place to maintain excellence in the future.

PEOPLE: OLD WORLD VS. NEW WORLD

As with the other skills, there are views you may currently have that don't fit the model anymore. The Old World conception of the doctor as untouchable and protected does damage in the New World, negatively impacting relationships, and severely hurting your chances for success and satisfaction. In the New World, being a doctor isn't about being a *lone healer*; instead, it's about teamwork, collaboration, and mentorship.

PEOPLE

OLD WORLD VIEWS	NEW WORLD VIEWS
I fight for what my patients need, no matter who loses in the process.	If anyone loses, we all lose — my patients can't win if I don't have support from administrators, nurses, and everyone else in my organization.
I listen to solve problems — if I don't have the answer, why am I part of the conversation?	I listen to build trust and understanding — not just to provide a magic solution.
I have credibility in my specialty, and that's all I need.	I need to be a credible resource for others in my organization when it comes to issues that affect the whole system, not just my specialty.
I'm a patient healer, and it's fine to limit my efforts to my patients — that's why I'm here.	It is my duty and responsibility to ensure my patients are served well into the future — which is why I must grow and develop others as well as growing and developing myself.

DISCUSSION: WIN-WIN, TRUST, CREDIBILITY, AND SUPPORT

The business literature about building effective relationships puts a variety of labels on the behaviors that are most important when dealing with others. But if you read enough of those books — and we certainly have — you start to see commonalities. At the end of the day, we believe it's a journey through four attributes: win-win, trust, credibility, and support. Each are unique, critical elements that build upon each other — and are necessary to thrive in the New World and be the leader (and team player) a rescued doctor needs to be.

WIN-WIN

If anyone comes away a loser, we have all lost, especially our patients.

As much as it doesn't always seem like it, the world is not zero-sum. If you win, it doesn't mean others have to lose. It all comes back to the *Enemies vs. Partners* trap we discussed earlier — the people around you are not your enemies when it comes to your patients; they're your partners, and all of you need to have the mindset that you're working together for the good of the entire patient population. What that means is that solutions where you come out ahead aren't actually wins if it means that other people are losing something in the process. Your new equipment is far less valuable if it means that three nurses are laid off and can't be there to help your patients. Instead, it's imperative to find solutions that create new value for everyone — what new programs, for instance, can be created to fund your new equipment so that staff doesn't have to be affected, and everyone can benefit?

Embracing the idea that everyone can win — that victories aren't in scarce supply and the best answer is one that works for all of the parties involved — is key to being a New World doctor. You're not in competition with the people around you. You're all after the same thing: quality care, provided within the limitations that are inevitable in any system. And in the long run, you and your patients lose if you aim for anything less than a win for everyone.

It's true that aiming for win-win doesn't mean that you will get your way every time. Your goals may not be the same as the goals of the people in the finance department who have to sign off on every expense. You want more time with your patients, or a costly new machine. You may not get that. But you need to come to the table with the idea that even if you don't get everything you're asking for, you should be able to find a solution that satisfies everyone's needs to enough of an extent that you can declare victory. If this is impossible — if you can't come up with an answer that helps everyone — you need to be willing to walk away. One side winning and one side losing is worse than no agreement at all. If you don't give yourself that option — if it's "everyone wins or we walk away" — then you will be forced to be think outside the box for new solutions that can end up being game-changers.

The truth is that when losing isn't an option — when everyone knows that you're playing for all sides to win — working together becomes much easier. You need to hear each other out and understand everyone's needs — and negotiate as partners looking for common ground instead of adversaries hoping to emerge victorious. It's not a battle, and when you all see yourself on the same side, new answers can present themselves, developed from everyone bringing their own expertise and skills to bear.

Too often, doctors disengage when they fear they won't get their way instead of deciding to work even harder. You can't disengage and still come out a winner. You need to search for opportunities. Otherwise, patients end up losing. Fundamentally, it's an intellectual choice. You can continue to compete, or you can drop the need to come out ahead and act instead for the good of all.

Once you have the win-win mindset — when people know you are out for everyone and not just for yourself — you can take huge leaps forward.

Knowing you are looking out for the entire system is the first step toward building real, authentic trust with your colleagues, so that they don't need to be skeptical of your motives or always wondering what your angle is.

TRUST

Trust can't be built without listening — listening to understand, not just solve a problem.

Inspiring trust in others, and behaving so that they truly believe that you are serious about change — that you mean what you say about making things better for everyone — is a huge part of what being a New World doctor is about. For a long time, doctors have been seen as there for their patients but not for the entire organization. For a rescued doctor, that isn't the case anymore. Being firmly in the New World means you're there for everyone. To take on the challenges of a rescued doctor, people have to be willing — eager — to work with you. Which means they have to trust you.

It's not like trust is a new skill for doctors to have. In the Old World, trust was the most important instrument for getting a patient to rely on you, to listen and follow through on his treatment plan, and to come back and see you again. It's obvious that trust is and has always been a given with patients. You can't be an effective doctor without it. But trust among all of the key stakeholders in your organization hasn't been seen as an equally important requirement. Too often, the drivers of New World medicine show themselves — seeing others as enemies instead of partners, disengaging when a situation is outside your specialty, ignoring the business concerns outside of medicine, or refusing to accept that it's part of a doctor's job to be involved in all of the issues of the hospital, not just the ones most directly about their patients. No one can trust you if they don't think you care about their concerns and are really listening, with the intent of acting and helping, instead of merely waiting to get back to your own silo and your own work.

It's not enough anymore, as you move from serving individuals to serving the entire system, to only be an advocate for yourself and your patients. You're not an effective patient advocate if no one is willing to support you, stand with you, and fight. Trust, despite what you may think, isn't something passive. It's active. You need to back up what you say with actual activity. You inspire trust because people not only believe you but believe *in* you. They believe you will fight for them and their agenda just like you want them to fight for you and yours. Trying to dictate to others may have worked (a little) in the Old World when doctors were feared and locked into the center of the system — but in the New World, it's not the way to get things done. Doctors, for better or worse, aren't feared anymore. They're either taking on the New World challenges or they're ignored, marginalized, worked around, and left on Doctor Island to fend for themselves. That's not where you want to be. That's why you're taking on this journey.

The key skill to build trust is listening. But not just listening to solve problems — listening to truly, genuinely understand. You can't build trust without hearing the people around you and what they're trying to communicate. But you need to listen not only as a specialist but also as a generalist. As a generalist, you don't need to solve everyone's problems. You need to comprehend their perspective — and have empathy. Doctors are used to listening to patients — but it's often a different kind of listening. We're talking here about listening without trying to come up with a differential diagnosis, listening without trying to cure, but listening to understand and see the challenges that someone is facing and listening to feel their frustrations and needs.

Beyond listening, you build trust by making (and then, of course, keeping) promises that can make a difference. How do you know what promises make a difference to someone? If you've really been listening, you'll know. You make the right promises, that matter to others and then you become a trusted partner in whatever they are trying to accomplish. An effective New World doctor will survey the entire landscape and look for opportunities to make a difference and become that trusted partner — volunteering to step up and involve themselves in causes important to the hospital or to their colleagues, using their particular skills in the service of others, building those relationships, inspiring trust, and gaining an army of colleagues who will, in turn, fight for the causes most important to them.

It's not only about responding when someone asks — it's about being proactive and seeking out the chance to help. Do that enough times, and with enough commitment, and you will have trust. In turn, once you have that trust developed, you move on to the next stage — credibility, or making sure that others realize you are not only someone who is on their side, but you are in fact able to add real and significant value to their fight.

CREDIBILITY

Understanding enough to create a whole greater than the sum of its parts.

As with listening and trust, credibility isn't something that's new to doctors — at least not when it comes to patients. As a clinician, credibility is self-evident — if you don't have credibility, patients simply aren't going to listen to you (and they shouldn't). But it's much the same in the broader generalist world of the hospital, even though that's a world many doctors have been ignoring for far too long. For you to make progress on your organizational goals, to harness the support of others, and to get them to fight for you and with you, it's crucial that you have credibility in their eyes, beyond just your clinical competence.

We're talking about credibility in the New World facets of the job, the activities that extend beyond the clinical. Of course you still need to be absolutely credible clinically as a New World doctor. But that is no longer enough. You now need credibility in the other arenas that have a presence in the New World. You need to have a basic understanding of how your organization works. You need to know enough about finance and business to be part of the conversation. You need to know your stakeholders and the issues that are pressing on your organization, the limitations they're up against, the opportunities that it's possible to pursue, and the goals that they're chasing — all of what we discussed when you were gaining clarity, plus the ideas and contributions that emerge when you actually sit down and think about these issues (as you must, as part of your Quadrant Two time).

None of this means you have to be an expert in the same way that you're an expert on the clinical side. You don't need to be an expert in business or have an MBA in order to contribute. In the generalist world, credibility is different than it is in medicine. You don't need to know all the research or have all the answers. You just need to know enough to be part of the conversation. Being a smart, engaged person doesn't get you a lot on the clinical side without medical training. You can't come up with a treatment plan if you've never gone to medical school. But the generalist world deals with problems we all think about as human beings living in the world. We can all have opinions about how to save money or how to decide between opportunities or how to make smart choices. With a little bit of knowledge about our organization, and a little bit of smart thinking, we can all be part of those discussions in a way that someone who isn't a trained doctor simply can't be when it comes to treatment decisions.

In this book, we're trying to make you fluent, or at least start that journey. We know that you can't, in 130 pages, become an expert in business or change management. But you don't need to be. It's not what the job requires. You just need to be more fluent than you were in the Old World, and understand that these issues are in fact worth your time and energy.

In the Old World, no one admits when they don't know something. The definition of credibility for a doctor is knowing the answer. If you don't know how to diagnose someone, if you don't know how the body works, you are not credible. But in the generalist world, you can spend two hours reading a book and know enough to productively attend a meeting and contribute some ideas. You have colleagues who are experts — or at least they should be — but they need your perspective as well. Experts in finance don't necessarily know the right priorities for doctors — and with just a little bit of understanding of what the finance experts are dealing with, you can be a tremendous resource to them as they figure out the right decisions to make.

What we're talking about, in a lot of ways, is synergy. Knowing enough to contribute makes it possible to work with the people throughout your organization — in finance, management, and elsewhere — and give them a bit of perspective that will help them make better decisions. By knowing enough to be able to engage, you help get to a solution that's better than they can achieve alone, and also better than you could achieve without the knowledge that they bring to the table. That's what synergy is: an outcome greater than the sum of its parts.

In medicine, you naturally protect your credibility. It's a huge issue, not wanting to make a mistake as a doctor. But in the generalist world — in business — it's all about making mistakes, testing hypotheses, and trial and error. You don't lose credibility by taking a risk the way you would in medicine. Business is all about taking risks. You have to take risks. No one knows for sure what will happen if you invest in one program over another, hire this person instead of that person, open one door instead of another. There isn't necessarily ever enough proof to fully justify the creation of a new department, a new clinic, a new program, without anyone being able to have doubts or ask questions. There is always some degree of uncertainty in the business world. You just want people to be comfortable relying on you for your thoughts and ideas, knowing and trusting that everyone ultimately wants the same outcome as you do — better health care for your patients.

There's one more piece when it comes to *People*. You may have the right win-win mentality, people may trust you, you may be someone they find credible enough to rely on, but even if all of those pieces are in place, it's not enough. It may be enough for now, but it's not enough for the future — yours or your patients'. The final piece is about taking other people on the journey with you, developing the talent around you at the same time that you are developing yourself.

SUPPORT
One rescued doctor can't change a hospital alone.

Growing and developing others is so critical to the Rescue The Doctor path, because it's so critical to what doctors need to do in the New World. In the Old World, it was okay to work in your own silo, see your own patients, rely on yourself and yourself alone. No more. No one is successful in the New World without a team — and teams don't just create themselves. The skills we're offering you are the skills you need to offer others — for their benefit, but also for yours. Rescuing yourself has to ultimately about more than just you, because the amount you can do alone is limited. One rescued doctor, no matter how gifted, can't change an entire hospital. It takes a team working together — with a win-win mindset, with trust, with credibility, but also with support, and by serving as models for each other and reinforcement when things become challenging. So much of the frustration of doctors right now is feeling alone — adrift on Doctor Island — without a team behind them, without common goals and a common purpose. Rescuing doctors is about building those teams and making your job about more than just yourself as a *lone healer*.

Being a New World doctor is about teaching and collaborating and carrying others on your shoulders. It's about identifying potential champions around you — on your team, in your organization, and in the broader world of health care — and encouraging them. It's about rescuing yourself by rescuing others — about experiencing the reward of being part of something larger than yourself. Doctors are fortunate in that you have spent all of history helping people through your work. It's what a doctor does. But, just as with trust and credibility, these efforts have all been patient-focused. It's just as important to turn inward and apply these ideas to the colleagues and stakeholders around you. You need to think about helping them too.

Truth is, the tangible reward of helping patients is disappearing for a lot of doctors in the New World. As medicine has become more fragmented, as patients have become shared among many doctors and not healed solely by one, much of the ownership over any particular patient is gone. In your specialist world, you don't always even know what happens to your patients. You don't get the satisfaction of seeing them healed or following their entire story. But in the New World you can get those rewards in the generalist world — you can see your entire institution healed, and you can be a key cog in improving the experience for all patients, not just a few of them. Through the generalist lens, you can make a difference — not just as a specialist.

This means mentoring others, taking time to be interested in the careers of the people around you, taking time to work with them on the same kinds of skills we've been developing in this book, taking time to listen to them and bring them onto your team. It means helping to rescue others, and letting others help rescue you. It means leading by example, and holding yourself out as someone others can turn to for guidance and for help. Rescuing others is the only way to truly rescue yourself.

* * *

The four skills we've just talked about — win-win, trust, credibility, and support — are purposely presented in that order. They build upon each other, like blocks being stacked in a tower. Your win-win mindset is the first thing you need. Only then can you start to build trust. And it is only once you have that trust that your credibility starts becoming a factor. Finally, with the right mindset, and with those around you trusting you and working with you, you are in a position to grow and develop others — to support your colleagues. Putting it all together, you are ready to *deliver*, and to make a real difference.

Frankly, it doesn't take that many doctors to make a noticeable difference — to a team, to an organization, to a hospital, to an entire health care system. Doctors are so critical that what each one does truly matters. If only a few doctors are rescued, and they each begin to rescue a few others, very quickly you gain a critical mass that can build a great health care system. That is what *delivery* is about — harnessing these skills you've picked up here, harnessing the power of just a few rescued doctors — and engineering transformative change, now and into the future. In the next section, we'll talk about what happens when you've mastered these skills and a rescued doctor is unleashed into the system — and what it means to deliver breakthrough health care in the New World.

DELIVER

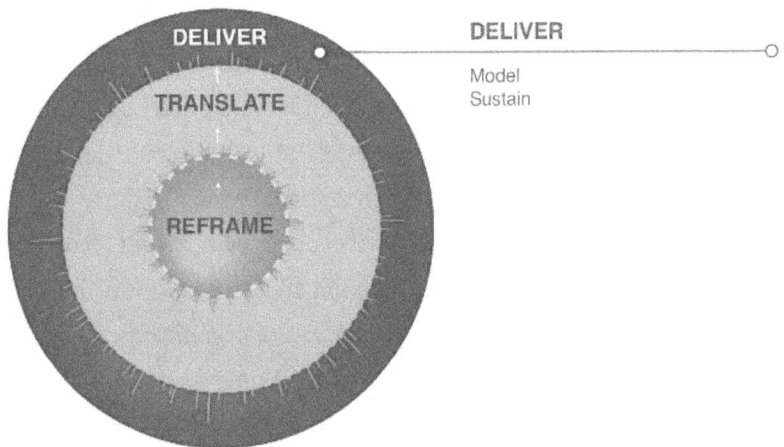

RESCUE THE DOCTOR

DELIVER

Model
Sustain

If you look at any group of people, there will always be some who stand out — who do things differently, who make things happen, who lead the people around them to improve life for everyone. We talked earlier about those colleagues who seem to have transcended the problems that doctors are facing, and are thriving in spite of the challenges. There is a concept known as Positive Deviance that focuses on paying attention to those people — the kinds of people who get exceptional, unusual results — and looking at how they behave, and then trying to replicate those behaviors throughout an organization. In doing so, the goal is to turn the outliers — the ones effectively blazing their own unique paths — into the mainstream.[26] These champions — who are already succeeding in the organization — become the role models for everyone else, and their behaviors help lead change from the inside out. As opposed to bringing outsiders in — who can never truly be accepted, especially in a field like medicine, which requires so much specialized knowledge and expertise that outsiders won't have — the Positive Deviance models are about helping those already on the inside to become agents of change and leaders for the entire organization.

In many ways, Rescue The Doctor is built on a model like this, except that those internal role models are, in many cases, yet to make themselves known. But if you truly take what you've learned in this book to heart, and use it to transform your professional life, we believe you can become exactly that role model, exactly that agent of change, exactly that leader who can help your organization triumph over the challenges facing health care and become a beacon of light for a health care future better than it is today.

Doctors are perfectly positioned to be the leaders — indeed, we hope we have made the case that doctors are the only ones perfectly positioned to lead. You have the expertise, you have the mission, and, now, we hope, you have the skills. We want you to become the positive deviants, the pioneers who return

---

[26] For more about positive deviance:
http://opinionator.blogs.nytimes.com/2013/02/27/when-deviants-do-good/

doctors to the center of health care and march us to a better tomorrow. Change that comes from the outside doesn't work — the experiences of so many doctors and hospitals bears that out — but change that comes from the inside, from the doctors themselves, can be truly transformative.

> *"Change artists come into town, offer their wisdom, collect their fees, and then head home, where they design more offerings, conduct more research, and pen more books. In a time of dizzying change, change programs are a growth industry. And not surprisingly, these change programs almost never work. The consultants decamp, and the company reverts to form. The book gets read, maybe even passed around, and the company reverts to form. The motivational speaker leaves to applause, and the company reverts to form."*[27]

* * *

We've spent over a hundred pages explaining the changes in health care that are making happy, fulfilling professional lives more and more challenging for doctors, and then, in the *translate* section, giving you the essentials you need to cope, change, and thrive even in this difficult environment. But understanding the landscape and knowing what you need to do are useless if you don't actually *deliver*.

It's not just about making your own life better — which is, of course, critical — but it's also about making the system better, making your colleagues better, and, ultimately, making your patient care far better than it can be in the current system. Once you have mastered the concepts in the *reframe* and *translate* sections of the book, you are ready — and it is your

---

[27] http://www.fastcompany.com/42075/positive-deviant

obligation — to *deliver*. Only then can you truly become rescued, rescue others, and rescue the system.

What does *delivery* mean? It means acting on the knowledge you've gained, and it means creating real, lasting change, from the inside. Too often it's outsiders being brought in — gurus from other industries, managers with business and finance experience in industries far afield from health care, or politicians and bureaucrats making decisions without having medical expertise. We firmly believe that especially in medicine, given the stakes and the complexity, doctors must be at the core.

For our Rescue The Doctor model, *delivery* has two parts:

MODEL

and

SUSTAIN

In a way, these two parts are like the micro- and macro- versions of *delivery*. Model is about the changes you make, on the ground, right now. Sustain is about making sure it lasts for the future — that the structure is changed for the better, the organization is secure, and you've built, in essence, a machine that can keep running even after you and your colleagues are gone.

Model is the Positive Deviance approach in action. You can't just take this new knowledge you've gained, put the book on your bookshelf, and go on living your life like you've been living it up until this point. You need to actually do things differently — and do them in a way that your colleagues can see, understand, and learn from. It is not enough to be the only rescued doctor in your institution — because then you're not truly rescued at all. For doctors to be rescued, the movement has to spread. You need to be a role model for your colleagues, you need to share the insights you've gained, and you need to all work together to rescue the system.

This doesn't mean that everyone has to go on this journey — there will always be people stuck in the Old World, stubbornly refusing to accept the reality that the clock will not be turning backwards. But there is a rule of thumb that, generally speaking, the number of people that must be involved in changing an organization is the square root of the number of people in the group itself. A group of a hundred can be changed by ten people; an organization of 10,000 can be changed by merely 100. These are the people you have to identify as leaders and the people you need to bring along on your journey toward rescue. In turn, they will find their own people to develop, and, eventually, the system will change.

But it can't stop there. Rescuing a handful of doctors is useless if the changes don't last. If we bring doctors back from Doctor Island, back to the center of health care, it would be a crushing blow if in the next generation they just start drifting away again, returning to the same kinds of Old World thinking that are paralyzing doctors now. We need to build a sustainable machine so that change lasts, and so that health care is truly made better, not just now but in the future.

That means we need to make it so that the lessons of Rescue The Doctor are brought to the youngest doctors, and made part of every doctor's education — starting in medical school (and, for those who have to work closely with doctors, as part of their education as well). As we have been saying, learning medicine is of course required but it is no longer enough on its own. An effective doctor in the New World needs to know more than just medicine — he needs to understand the generalist world of business, he needs to understand human relationships and mentorship and collaboration. He needs to be a team player and a system healer — and that's difficult when all that is currently taught is how to be a healer of individual patients, alone, in your own separate silo.

No matter what the future of health care holds, doctors must be prepared with these skills, prepared and ready to meet the challenges, and not just sitting on the sidelines, letting others make the decisions and hoping for the best. Doctors need to be the ones leading, not following — acting, not *re*acting.

* * *

Part of the mission we talked about at the beginning of the *translate* section involved investing in yourself, making the commitment to go on this journey and truly change. Just as critical to that mission is understanding that you need to leave a legacy. It is the responsibility of every doctor — if he truly cares about his patients and their future — to ensure that the profession is well-positioned to continue providing the best possible care going forward, even after you are no longer practicing. Leaving that legacy means developing others, mentoring, leading, sharing the lessons you've learned with your colleagues and the rest of your team. It means putting in place systems to ensure that change continues, whether it's check-ins or meetings or status updates. You need to prevent people — yourself and others — from drifting back into complacency and once again ending up burned out and disaffected. You need to create sustainable change, sustainable leadership (medical and otherwise) at all levels, a system that is not just changed but transformed.

Delivery means all of this — because what you get when you effectively deliver is something far beyond what you have now. You get fulfillment, satisfaction, reward — and your patients in turn get fulfilled and satisfied doctors who are truly serving them the best that they can be served. You get reminded every day of why you chose this profession, and why it's a profession that, until recently, has always been held in the utmost esteem by society. You get back your career — your calling — instead of just having a job. And you get back your pride in being a doctor, and practicing the best medicine you can.

You have a choice: you can accept change that is forced upon you, or you can take the lead yourselves. Those are the options. You have the choice.

* * *

You may not have expected, when you started reading this book, to finish it feeling like we've thrown even more responsibilities onto your plate than you had when you began. You probably thought we would just be giving you some time management techniques, telling you how to stand up to the 'enemies' in business, finance, and elsewhere trying to tell you how to practice medicine, and urging you to fight for the areas of decision-making that should rightly belong to doctors and shouldn't be snatched away.

Instead, we're telling you that your entire way of thinking about being a doctor has to change. We're telling you that you need to work even more with the people around you than you're already being forced to. We're telling you that you have to mentor others, get involved in your institution, be a leader — when all you wanted was another hour of sleep each night and not having to feel like your decision to go to medical school was a mistake.

But there are no quick fixes, and, we promise you — the kind of change we are trying to inspire will truly make a difference for you, and for health care. The problems doctors are struggling with — burnout, frustration, lack of control — are not inevitable. Things can and will get better if doctors move from the Old World to the New World and embrace the opportunity to lead. The New World doctor sees the world differently. He understands the system, and the forces at work that are impacting his career. He sees his colleagues not as enemies but as partners. He recognizes that medicine and business can no longer be separate. He realizes that he needs to think not only like a specialist but also like a generalist. And he accepts that what makes a good doctor is different than what it used to be.

In the New World, the fog has lifted. Doctors are back in control, helping to influence and lead their organizations and shape their profession.

They do not have to be on the sidelines. *You do not have to be on the sidelines.*

Picture the doctor you can be, once you follow through on the steps in this book and become truly rescued. You walk in the doors of your hospital ready for the day, not despondent to be there. You have an agenda, and it's an agenda you care about. You have colleagues and stakeholders who respect you, understand you, seek you out for guidance and advice — and in turn you have colleagues and stakeholders you respect and understand, who you can turn to for help.

Patients notice the difference. They see a calmer, less restless doctor, more dedicated, more focused. Others certainly notice the difference. They see you as someone on their side, someone they don't have to be afraid to approach. Someone who approaches them. Not as an opponent but as a team player, trying to understand and hoping to contribute. Knowing that everyone needs to work together if patients are going to be helped.

In this environment, management certainly isn't pushing the doctor aside, instituting policies despite what doctors want, acting to command and control. Instead, management is recognizing that doctors are indeed back at the center of the model, an integral part of the system with the power to bring their colleagues along.

The Old World was static, every day the same. The New World has movement. Problems are addressed, things are getting better. If you open the door of that New World hospital, *doctors* are at the head of the meeting tables, feeling the responsibility to heal the organization, and empowered enough to do it. Ambitions in the New World go beyond just patient care. How can you be more than just another hospital — how can you serve your patients better, differently, optimally?

We have given you the skills to start. It is up to you to rescue yourself, rescue your colleagues, and rescue health care. We know you're up for the challenge, because otherwise you never would have picked up this book. As an exercise, here at the end, try to picture yourself as a fully rescued doctor — in charge of your career, making a difference, inspiring others, and leading the way. Picture what that doctor looks like, try to see him or her from every angle, and imagine what it would feel like to have gotten yourself to that place — in your organization, and in your career. Know that you can become that doctor — we assure you that it is entirely within your ability to do so.

A final note: we want to help you on your journey, however we can. Go to www.rescuethedoctor.com to share your experiences, and connect with us and other doctors around the world on the road to rescue. We can change health care, together, and rescue doctors, hospitals, and patients worldwide.

ABOUT THE AUTHORS

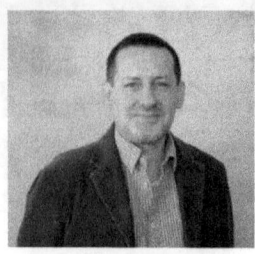

Dr. Peter P. Pramstaller, M.D., is a neurologist at the Central Hospital of Bolzano (Northern Italy), as well as the founding director and scientific head of the Center for Biomedicine at the European Academy (EURAC) of Bolzano and Associate Professor of Neurology at the Medical University of Luebeck (Germany). He lives with his wife and two children in St. Pauls/Eppan, just outside Bolzano.

Matt Smith is a Director of Beffective, an award-winning organization helping hospitals improve their performance. For the past eighteen years, Matt has also been a senior international consultant with Franklin Covey, working with large multi-national organizations. He lives with his wife and two children on the Isle of Wight (UK).

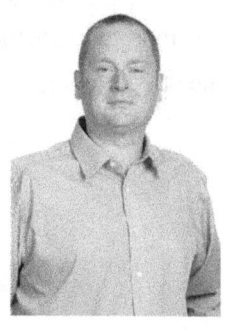

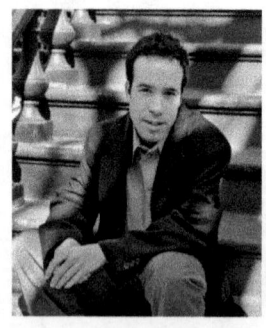

Jeremy Blachman is a writer for print, film, and television, based in the U.S. A graduate of Harvard Law School, he is the author of *Anonymous Lawyer* (Henry Holt), a novel satirizing the world of corporate law, developed for television in the United States by Sony and NBC and published in seven languages around the world. He lives with his wife (a medical doctor) and son in New York.

www.ingramcontent.com/pod-product-compliance
Lightning Source LLC
Chambersburg PA
CBHW051720170526
45167CB00002B/740